RESOURCE ALLOCATION
IN THE HEALTH SERVICE
A review of the methods of the
Resource Allocation Working Party (RAWP)

RESOURCE ALLOCATION IN THE HEALTH SERVICE
A review of the methods of the Resource Allocation Working Party (RAWP)

Nicholas Mays
Gwyn Bevan

Bedford Square Press | NCVO

First published 1987 by the
Bedford Square Press of the
National Council for Voluntary Organisations
26 Bedford Square
London WC1B 3HU

© 1987 Social Administration Research Trust

ISBN 0 7199 1192 3

Printed in Great Britain by Antony Rowe Ltd, Chippenham

Series Foreword

This series of Occasional Papers was started in 1960 to supply the need for a medium of publication for studies in the field of social policy and administration which fell between the two extremes of the short article and the full-length book. Since the inception of this Series of papers, it has, however, been extended to include many which might better be described as books: comparative speed of publication being one factor that has attracted authors to us. It was thought that such a series would not only meet a need among research workers and writers concerned with contemporary social issues, but would also strengthen links between students of the subject and administrators, social workers, committee members and others with responsibilities and interest in the social services.

Contributions to the series are welcome from any source and should be submitted in the first instance to the Secretary, Social Administration Research Trust at the London School of Economics, Houghton Street, London WC2A 2AE.

The series is now published by the Bedford Square Press to which all queries about this and previous titles should be addressed.

Contents

ACKNOWLEDGEMENTS

This book began life as a literature review on RAWP commissioned by the Department of Health and Social Security from the Social Medicine and Health Services Research Unit at St Thomas' Hospital and undertaken by Nicholas Mays. We are grateful to DHSS for their financial support to the Research Unit. However, the authors alone are responsible for the views contained in this book. We should particularly like to thank John Smith who was the Chairman of RAWP, 1975-76, for his kindness in contributing a preface and for his valuable comments and observations on various chapters of the draft. We found our discussions with him fascinating and immensley helpful in understanding the context within which RAWP emerged. A number of other people have provided help, advice and encouragement over the last two years, particularly Professor Brian Abel-Smith, Cliff Graham and Professor Peter Townsend. A number of our colleagues in the Department of Community Medicine have given up large amounts of time to read sections of the manuscript in a spirit of constructive criticism, particularly John Brazier, Walter Holland, Roger Beech, Myfanwy Morgan and Marian Craig. Carolyn Green, with the help of Kate Redmond and Yvonne Smith has borne the brunt of the word-processing. We are very grateful to them and to all the other secretarial staff in the Department of Community Medicine, particularly in the latter stages to Nicky Smith, who have helped out with parts of the manuscript at different times.

The book is the result of close collaboration between the two authors over a two year period. In terms of original authorship, Chapters One to Seven were written by Nicholas Mays and Chapter Eight by Gwyn Bevan.

Nicholas Mays
Gwyn Bevan

December 1986

PREFACE

It is often remarked that attitudes towards RAWP are coloured by its effect upon the perceived interests of the observer. Certainly much effort has been devoted to seeking weaknesses in its recommended methodology which might be exploited to the advantage - or perhaps to the lesser disadvantage - of interests which have imagined themselves threatened by its impact.

In this comprehensive and illuminating review of the literature inspired by RAWP over a decade, Nicholas Mays and Gwyn Bevan exhibit a refreshing objectivity. They have sought to uncover and elaborate the thinking and reasoning underlying RAWP's recommendations before attempting any judgement as to whether the conclusions were soundly based at the time or whether, with hindsight, they might now be questioned. I can pay no greater compliment to their objectivity than to observe that when reading their book I have on occasion been uncannily reminded of the debates which attended the deliberations of my colleagues and myself when we grappled with the issues during that long hot summer of 1976. The weather may be different but the issues remain largely unchanged.

This review performs an invaluable service. It rehearses the major issues in depth and painstakingly sets them in their right context. This is a welcome departure from much earlier commentary. At the same time, as a collation and distillation of views on a broad front, it provides a foundation for the exploration of some more recent ideas.

A Preface is not the place to express a personal view either on the conclusions which the authors reach or the aspects which they judge would profit from further research and study. But perhaps I may be permitted a final conclusion.

The authors rightly draw attention to the importance of making a proper distinction between those programmes which have a direct bearing on the social environment, eg. housing, employment opportunity, financial support etc. and, per contra, health care programmes which have to treat the consequences in terms of ill health of any failures in maintaining an acceptable social environment. A Joint Approach to Social Policy seems as necessary today as it was a decade ago. Hopefully this will not be overlooked when issues identified as worthy of further examination in the health care field alone, come to be considered.

J.C.C. Smith
(Chairman of the Resource Allocation Working Party 1975-1976)
Whitchurch Hill
Oxfordshire

November 1986

CHAPTER ONE

INTRODUCTION

In April 1986 the Chairman of the National Health Service (NHS) Management Board within the Department of Health and Social Security (DHSS) announced a review of the operation of the Resource Allocation Working Party (RAWP) formula. The review is scheduled to report at the end of 1986, or early 1987, 'with proposals for improving the way in which the national RAWP formula measures relative need for the hospital and community health services, taking account of .... work carried out on modifications to the RAWP formula at sub-regional level,'... (DHSS, 1986a). The aim of this book is to draw together the scattered threads of the extensive literature surrounding RAWP and thus, to contribute to the debate which has continued ever since the original RAWP report of 1976 to establish the best method of allocating NHS financial resources fairly between different parts of England. This debate is sure to quicken when the results of the Management Board's review are published.

From its inception in 1948 until 1976, the NHS was funded on the basis of existing levels of activity with annual increases for growth and developments when economic circumstances permitted. The implementation of the report of the Resource Allocation Working Party marked a decisive, radical shift to capitation-based finance on the basis of need (DHSS, 1976c). Similar resource allocation formulae based on population need were devised and implemented in Wales, Scotland and Northern Ireland. John Carrier described RAWP at the time as, 'the most significant attempt at planned change in the NHS (not withstanding the 1974 reorganisation) since its inception in 1948' (Carrier, 1978, p.120). RAWP aimed 'to secure, through resource allocation, that there would eventually be equal opportunity of access to health care for people at equal risk' (DHSS, 1976c, p.7, para. 1.3). With such an objective it is no surprise that the RAWP method has been the subject of extensive criticism and controversy ever since it was first implemented in 1977/78. However, the underlying principle of equity in the availability of health service resources has not been challenged and RAWP has remained in place through both Labour and Conservative administrations. RAWP is significant, therefore, not only because its methods shape the long-term distribution of millions of pounds of NHS resources, but also because of its longevity. The rationale and principles for reallocation developed in only fourteen months by an ad hoc working party of NHS officers, DHSS civil servants and academics have survived relatively unscathed through a decade of major political upheaval and economic deterioration. The Working Party had to work quickly and was given a daunting remit which would have reduced many groups to impotence:

'"To review the arrangements for distributing NHS capital and revenue to RHAs, AHAs and Districts respectively with a view to establishing a method of securing, as soon as practicable, a pattern of distribution responsive objectively, equitably and efficiently to relative need and to make recommendations."'
(DHSS, 1976c, p.5)

RAWP had to make the best of the available data. Yet its recommendations were rapidly implemented and have continued to guide DHSS resource allocation to Regions, almost unchanged. Below Regional level, Regions have to varying degrees modified the original RAWP methods. Unlike so many attempts at rational planning in government, RAWP has been a qualified success. It represents perhaps the most sophisticated and objective system in the world for establishing the fair share of health service resources to which each administrative population is entitled.

When the RAWP formula was first applied to the NHS budget in 1977/78 there was a 27% difference in expenditure in relation to need between the poorest and the wealthiest NHS Regions (Winyard, 1981). After almost ten years of gradual redistribution, the gap between the best-off and the least well-provided Region has narrowed substantially. It is expected that at the end of 1986/87 all Regions with the exception of North East Thames and North West Thames (the two most 'over-target' Regions), will be within 4% of their RAWP revenue 'target' income (Birch and Maynard, 1986). Thus, at Regional level, despite problems caused by the sluggish rate of growth in overall NHS resorces and the initial reluctance of DHSS to reduce the budgets of the over-target Regions in real terms, substantial progress towards RAWP 'targets' has been achieved. Regional 'targets' have been calculated on a reasonably consistent basis over the period and the gap between RHA current expenditure and future 'target' has generally narrowed each year although the pace of movement to target has varied widely between Regions. However, sub-Regionally, where the reliability of RAWP 'targets' is more questionable and where RHAs have used a variety of modified RAWP methods for setting resource 'targets', inequalities in resource availability and use were much greater at the beginning of the RAWP process and as a result, very marked inequalities remain (DHSS, 1985a). Even among the Districts with teaching hospitals which are generally regarded as the best provided in each Region, the variation in expenditure in relation to population is striking. In 1984/85, the cost of the use of acute inpatient services per capita by the residents of Paddington and North Kensington District, allowing for the age/sex structure and morbidity of the population was 197% of the national average. The equivalent figure for Nottingham, the lowest spending, teaching District was 92% of the national average. The range of acute inpatient expenditure for all Districts lay between Paddington and North Kensington, 197% and Chichester, 70% of the national average (DHSS, 1986b). At the sub-Regional level, redistribution has now to be financed by reductions in the allocations of the over-target Districts because of the restricted level of growth in the NHS budget nationally. It is inevitable that this will mean the provision of a lower level of services in the over-target Districts. This has been resisted by these loser Districts particularly in inner London, with the result that the four Thames Regions which are the best-provided and where the problem of sub-Regional redistribution is most severe, have been kept above their RAWP targets.

RAWP methods provide a reasonable way of establishing the resource entitlements of Regions, since at this level, with populations of several millions, it is relatively straightforward to relate expenditure to the population served. However, sub-Regionally, where populations are far less homogeneous and where patient flows across administrative boundaries are of much greater significance, particularly in the conurbations, conventional RAWP targets work far less well as a means of setting achievable objectives for Districts. There are two major problems in applying RAWP sub-Regionally: the difficulty of linking the resource allocation process to the development and implementation of plans for services; and the limited control which District managers can exercise over the nature and pattern of patient flows into and especially out of Districts. In response to these problems, a number of potential alternatives to a capitation-based formula have been put forward for use sub-Regionally. In broad terms, two contrasting solutions have been put forward; one based on the elaboration of Regional strategic planning; and the other based on the use of quasi-market mechanisms, such as cross-charging. These two very different approaches represent the emergence in Great Britain of the longstanding debate in many other health care systems between those who would wish to fund health services fairly for what they do and those who wish to fund health services fairly on the basis of the needs of the populations they serve. Quasi-market solutions rely on the incentives generated by a competitive environment to secure an equitable distribution of efficient health services. The planning-based solutions rely on the assumption that rational plans initiated by Regional Health Authorities (RHAs) can be negotiated, agreed and implemented by Districts, despite the fact that some will lose and some will gain in the process of redistribution.

RAWP has attracted an extensive literature of criticism and comment. Much of it is narrowly technical. The review which follows does not attempt to be exhaustive, but aims to discuss the issues which appear to the authors to be important, either because they touch on fundamental principles of equitable resource allocation, or because they are likely to affect the sums of money allocated to health authorities in a significant way, or because they have appeared in the terms of reference of the NHS Management Board review of RAWP. For example, the oft-voiced issue of the adequacy of the Service Increment for Teaching (SIFT), the allowance in the RAWP formula for the additional service costs incurred through the teaching of clinical medical and dental students, is not discussed in detail as a separate topic. A full assessment of the SIFT allowance has already been published elsewhere by one of the authors (Bevan, 1982b). The more general theme of the funding of teaching hospitals and the potential conflict between an equitable distribution of services and the beds and cases required for the clinical training of medical students, is discussed in Chapter Seven ('RAWP and Planning') and in the concluding chapter. Two major, long-term policy issues which RAWP was unable to tackle are likewise not given extended, separate treatment: the unequal distribution of Health Service expenditure between the different parts of the United Kingdom; and the relationship between the geographical distribution of District Health Authority hospital and community health services' expenditure covered by RAWP, and the distribution of Family Practitioner Committee (FPC) expenditure which lies outside the RAWP process. Both issues have recently been rehearsed by Birch and Maynard (1986)*. Whatever the intrinsic merits of the arguments for reform in both cases, political reality points in the opposite direction. It is noteworthy that neither "UK RAWP" nor the integration of FPC and hospital and community health services' resource allocation featured in the list of topics on which the NHS Management Board sought comments during its recent review of national RAWP (DHSS, 1986a).

The book begins by setting RAWP in the context of NHS geographical resource allocation policy since 1948 (Chapter Two). There is more to this than mere antiquarian interest. Initiatives such as the 1962 Hospital Plan, although currently unfashionable in NHS circles, bear reinspection today. The contemporary relevance of an approach based on equalising the availability of capital stock is taken up in the concluding chapter (Chapter Eight). Furthermore, understanding a little more of the immediate context and manner in which RAWP was set up may go some way towards explaining its relative success and longevity. Part I, 'The Population and Population Weightings' considers the principal elements which contribute to the construction of RAWP targets as measures of the relative needs of populations. The focus is on how adequately

---

* They are also covered, along with a number of other issues, such as RAWP and the private sector, in a lengthier, unpublished review of the RAWP literature prepared by one of the authors (Mays).

population size, adjusted for cross-boundary flows, age/sex structure and a proxy allowance for further morbidity differences in the shape of standardised mortality ratios (SMRs), account for the relative health care resource needs of populations at Regional and sub-Regional levels. Particular attention is given to the controversy over the use of SMRs (Chapter Four) and the question of whether allowance should be made for social deprivation in RAWP (Chapter Five). While Part One concentrates on the measurement of population need for resource allocation purposes, Part Two considers the implications sub-Regionally of using the resultant RAWP targets to attempt to move from the current inequitable distribution of services towards a fairer future pattern. It is found that conventional RAWP methods are insufficiently integrated with the process of planning the future pattern of services to provide a helpful guide to the actions which Regions and Districts must take together to move toward equity. Chapter Six ('Managing Cross-Boundary Flows of Patients and the Pursuit of Equity') discusses quasi-market solutions to these problems of sub-Regional RAWP, while Chapter Seven ('RAWP and Planning') looks at a very different approach based on the strategic management of equity by RHAs. Chapter Eight attempts to pull together the three main themes of the book: measuring population need for health care resources; the merits of quasi-market mechanisms for securing equity; and the potential of Regional strategic management; as well as suggesting directions for future research.

CHAPTER TWO

THE ORIGINS OF RAWP: RESOURCE ALLOCATION BEFORE 1976

INTRODUCTION: THE OBJECTIVES OF THE NHS

In this chapter the intention is to place RAWP in its historical context with a brief account of spatial resource allocation policies and problems in the Health Service and their impact before 1976. This leads into a discussion of the circumstances surrounding the establishment of the Working Party and the main features of the environment in which it had to operate. It demonstrates two main features. Firstly, interest in equality of access to health services was not conspicuous before RAWP, particularly not in the 1950s. Secondly, the notion of normative planning with a view to providing a desirable range of provision for a population gained ground during the 1950s and 1960s to be replaced gradually in the 1970s by an approach based on rationing in response to economic stringency (Klein, 1983).

The 1944 White Paper which set out the wartime coalition government's intention to establish a National Health Service included the following high-flown statement:

> 'The Government...want to ensure that in the future every man and woman and child can rely on getting...the best medical and other facilities available; that their getting them shall not depend on whether they can pay for them or on any other factor irrelevant to real need.' (Ministry of Health, 1944, p.5)

And again, the 1946 Act promised a system which would be:

> 'available to everyone regardless of financial means, age, sex, employment or vocation, area of residence or insurance qualification.' (Ministry of Health, 1946)

These were very vague statements but they carried the logical implication that eventually policies would be devised to equalise the geographical distribution of resources (Culyer, Maynard and Williams, 1981). In the event, detailed policies for translating them into action were not forthcoming for 20 years. Maynard and Ludbrook (1980a) maintain that since the objectives of the NHS were not made explicit 'most discussion of their nature has been based on post hoc rationalizations...' They observe in a later piece that:

> '...when the Labour Party founded the new service on the basis of equal access for equal need, it might be more correct to interpret this as the principle that determined the form of the NHS (tax financed, universal coverage and no charges to patients) rather than as an objective that it was thought necessary to pursue actively.' (Maynard and Ludbrook, 1982, p. 109)

It seems that the prime consideration of the founders of the Health Service was to remove <u>financial</u> constraints on access to the existing pattern of health services, despite the fact that the NHS started with an unequal distribution of provision. There was little concern about remedying spatial inequalities in resources so long as there was freedom of access to what was available in each locality. There was certainly nothing in the NHS Act itself which would have brought about equality of availability, access, use or outcome (Cooper and Culyer, 1972).

The service was based on a number of other assumptions which have been rendered increasingly inappropriate by subsequent events. The two most important for this discussion were; firstly, that expenditure on the Service would not increase as the population was made healthier by its new-found access to free, modern, health care; and secondly, that there was therefore no need for policies and devices to ration financial and other resources and establish priorities. The early queues would eventually go away and there would be no need to resolve any competition for resources consistent with the objective of equal opportunity of access. Those responsible for setting up the Service were not in a position to foresee the great changes in medical technology, drug therapies, public expectations and disease burdens which have fundamentally altered both the supply and demand for health care since 1948.

RESOURCE ALLOCATION POLICIES, 1948-1962

NHS Resource allocation policies and their effects throughout the period up to 1980 have been summarised by Maynard and Ludbrook (1980 a).

During the period 1948-62 and especially in the 1950s, the principal concern of financial policy-makers in the Ministry of Health was to contain the increasing cost of the Health Service. Planning and funding of capital and revenue were largely incremental and <u>ad hoc</u> in character and the Regional resource inequalities which the Service had inherited in 1948 were not perceived as an important policy problem. As a result there was no explicit, public policy to reduce inequalities in resource distribution and they were little changed in the period. There is evidence that in certain respects (eg manpower) they were reinforced.

On the capital side, the hospital stock in 1948 was characterised by a lack of coordination, with large geographical differences in the distribution of beds. It was furthermore in poor condition (Nuffield Provincial Hospitals Trust, 1946). 45% of the hospitals had been built before 1891 and 21% before 1861 (Committee of Enquiry into the Cost of the National Health Service, 1956). However, the low level of capital investment in the 1950s (Government had put a higher priority on rebuilding industry, housing and schools) resulted in almost no new hospitals being built before 1962, although numbers of medical and nursing staff increased (Bennett and Holland, 1977). Such capital as there was (approximately £ 9 million during the period 1949-55 and an increasing amount in the period 1956-61) went on improving the efficiency of existing, antiquated hospitals through small schemes, rather than providing for parts of the country which needed new hospitals (Ministry of Health, 1962,p.1). In fact the overall quality of the hospital building stock declined and there is evidence that a relatively large proportion of the new investment in proportion to the needs of the rest of the country went on teaching hospitals schemes, especially in London. According to Smith (1984) 12% of the value of all capital schemes, 1955-62, went to London teaching hospitals. Such an outcome is unsurprising given the method of capital allocation. A central reserve was maintained for very large schemes. The capital allocation to Regional Hospital Boards (RHBs) was calculated mainly on the basis of population, whereas the Boards of

Governors of the teaching hospitals negotiated an allocation unrelated to population served, directly with the Ministry. Members of the Boards of Governors were also well represented in the House of Lords! Furthermore, the teaching hospitals in London were able to argue a case based on immediate need since their old buildings were in poor condition and this effectively closed off the option of long-term planning to help the areas without hospitals (Klein 1983, p. 53). This was exacerbated by the fact that only 5% of the national capital sum was reserved for RHBs in special need. Thus the distribution of major capital remained virtually unchanged geographically such that there was a failure to adapt allocations to reflect even the grossest changes in the location of the population (Lee, 1982). The distribution in favour of London teaching hospitals was reinforced by the existence of substantial voluntary funds administered by the Trustees of each of the ancient foundations. These funds were used to bolster public rebuilding programmes.

Revenue budgets were prepared by the Hospital Management Committees (HMCs) on the principle of maintaining previous levels of expenditure with a supplement to meet agreed 'urgent developments and improvements'. Increments tended to go to the noisiest rather than the neediest with no real review of previous activities, reflecting the prevailing power and influence structure of the NHS. Perhaps unkindly, Maynard and Ludbrook (1980a, p.293) encapsulated the process in the slogan:

"What you got last year, plus an allowance for growth, plus an allowance for scandals".

Hospital budgets were submitted by HMCs to the relevant Regional Hospital Board (RHB) which pulled their claims together into a Regional bid to the Ministry. The total NHS budget for the year was then divided among the RHBs in proportion to their expenditure in the last year for which figures were available. The RHBs then distributed resources to the HMCs in two parts (reflecting the structure of the original HMCs' Budgets): 1. the current costs of new developments and improvements - divided up partly on the basis of population and partly according to the capital projects likely to come onto operation during the financial year; and 2. the maintenance of existing services.

The criteria for the selection of capital developments by the Ministry (for large schemes) and by the RHBs (for smaller schemes) made little use of epidemiological data on population needs. The focus was on the need for immediate improvements to worn-out buildings. The method was very imprecise and as a result in the period 1957-70 the NHS budget grew at an annual rate of more than 4% per year without there being any sense of a national objective and steering mechanism. Only infrequently was an attempt made to assess the size of the budget in relation to the level of service provided.

Since allocations of both capital and revenue before 1970 depended on bidding processes, the quality of the case put forward by an authority was important as well as the amount of "noise" the authority could create and its political influence. The Boards of Governors of the teaching hospitals tended to attract a higher calibre of members than the HMCs and their administrators tended to be among the most able in the country. It is not surprising that members and officers were able to mount skilful and well argued cases for more money.

The rising cost of the Service in the 1950s and claims of extravagance prompted the Conservative Minister of Health Iain Macleod, to set up a committee of enquiry under C W Guillebaud to recommend means by which costs might be contained. The Committee's research staff were Richard Titmuss, Professor of Social Administration at the London School of Economics and Brian Abel-Smith, then a young Cambridge economist; later to become Senior Adviser to three labour Secretaries of State for Social Services, Richard Crossman (1968-70), Barbara

Castle (1974-76) and David Ennals (1976-79). In its report, the Committee was critical of the current system of allocating revenue funds for lacking 'a consistent long term objective'. Prompted by its researchers, the Committee considered the use of a resource allocation formula based on population need, but was forced to reject the idea on the grounds that 'any national formula would have to be weighted to take account of such a wide range of variables in Hospital Regions that it cannot be considered as a practical proposition at least for the present.' (Committee of Enquiry into the Cost of the National Health Service, 1956, p.104, para. 282). The Committee recognised the fundamental problem which continues to dog the RAWP approach of how to relate hospital activity to geographical populations, given that:

> 'Hospital Regions do not necessarily represent the "catchment areas" for the hospitals in their areas, and may take a large number of patients from adjoining Regions.' (Committee of Enquiry into the Cost of the National Health Service, 1956, p. 104, para. 282)

The Committee also noted the now familiar problem of allowing fairly for differences in hospital costs in a uniform formula. Although the Guillebaud Committee was unable to recommend a resource allocation formula, one of the researchers who had suggest it, Brian Abel-Smith, had ample opportunity subsequently, to plant the idea in the minds of Labour Ministers and DHSS civil servants.

The Committee's prinicipal conclusion on the NHS overall was that when the increasing volume of services provided was taken into account, the NHS was not becoming more costly. However, the current rate of hospital capital expenditure was inadequate and would damage the hospital service if allowed to continue.

The only explicit redistributive policy in this period concerned the geographical distribution of GPs. There were certain Ministry guidelines for hosptal resource distribution used by civil servants to try to favour "deprived" RHBs where this was possible, but it is doubtful if these had a great effect on the pattern of allocations. The setting up in 1948 of a Medical Practices Committee at Ministry level charged with ensuring 'adequate' numbers of GPs in each area of the country through the power to exclude practitioners from 'over-doctored' areas and the introduction in 1952 of a scheme of 'restricted' and 'designated' areas based on list sizes with related allowances had a limited effect in equalising the presence of GPs between different parts of the country (Butler, Bevan,and Taylor, 1973).

RESOURCE ALLOCATION POLICIES, 1962-1970

The first major, comprehensive attempt to link planning to resource allocation and explicitly to improve and ultimately remove the disparities in hospital resources in a strategic way, was the 1962 Hospital Plan for England and Wales (Ministry of Health, 1962) which set out an ambitious programme to spend more than £700 million at 1962 prices between 1962 and 1972 and a further £250 million between 1971 and 1975 (Smith, 1984). The proponents of the Plan were aware of the engrained geographical variation in provision (Ministry of Health, 1962, p.3) and aimed to modernise and rationalise the decaying hospital stock and make acceptable standards of provision (expressed in terms of bed:population ratios or 'norms' for acute and various non-acute specialties) available in all parts of England and Wales. The Hospital Plan thus aimed at equalisation through capital planning rather than direct revenue redistribution. Revenue increments were to follow capital schemes through the process known as RCCS (Revenue Consequences of Capital Schemes). This policy did have the potential to redistribute resources more equitably but only if the capital programme was assembled with the aim of securing equity. The Plan took no account of the fact

that per capita provision of euqal resources did not ensure euqal standards of
health care and health, since different parts of the country varied in their
levels of efficiency of resource use and in their health needs.

Allen (1981) has analysed the origins and formulation of the Plan in some detail
and concluded that the political decision to build hospitals came first, while
the rational enunciation of principles and norms and the development into a plan
came last. In this sense the Plan was another example of incrementalism and ex
post facto rationalisation rather than a radical change of approach.   Allen
(1981) explains the genesis of the Plan in 1962 in terms of :

1. the Guillebaud Committee's conclusion that the Health Service was
    neglecting capital investment to a dangerous extent;

2. studies of inequalities in Regional bed: population ratios and variations
    in efficiency, suggesting that there was some scope for equalisation and an
    overall reduction in the number of hospital beds;

3. changes in medical practice leading to professional pressure for new
    premises;

4. the improved state of the economy allowing both main political parties to
    espouse expansionary policies in the public sector;

5. energetic support for the Plan by Enoch Powell, Minister of Health and
    Bruce Fraser, Permanent Secretary at the Ministry of health.

The 1962 Plan was revised in the 1966 Hospital Building Programme which restated
the basic principles and bed norms of 1962, but essentially downgraded the
original intentions of the Plan. The equitable distribution of capital had to
be postponed in recognition of the fact that insufficient resources had been
made available up to 1966 and insufficient were likely to be available in the
future, to fund a transition to an equitable distribution within a decade
(Ministry of Health, 1966). The 1962 Plan had underestimated future health
needs and the costs of achieving its targets, and public expenditure cuts had
hampered its implementation. The 1966 Programme aimed to establish a common,
satisfactory standard of service but gave no timetable for this (Maynard and
Ludbrook, 1982).

Under the RCCS scheme, hospital revenue was distributed to meet the cost of new
hospital building. This benefited the Regions which had managerial skills to
make the most convincing cases for capital investment and the technical skills
to implement schemes swiftly. In England this was unlikely to favour the less
well-provided RHBs. Any further money which was available after RCCS, was used
to enable HMCs to make improvements. Larger proportionate shares were given to
those authorities whose needs seemed to be greatest. However, in reality there
was relatively little money left over to try and help the less well-provided
parts of the country. One contributory reason for this was the fact that under
RCCS there were no incentives for new hospitals to reduce their running costs or
to minimise the cost of schemes. As a result new hospitals tended to soak up
the available resources. Nevertheless, the DHSS produced evidence to the House
of Commons Expenditure Committee in 1971 showing that there had been some
gradual movement towards a fairer distribution of revenue. The range of per
capita revenue allocations to RHBs had narrowed in the period 1950/51 to 1971/72
(Abel-Smith, 1978). However, DHSS officials admitted that the revenue
allocation process 'was ... a somewhat subjective one' (House of Commons
Expenditure Committee, quoted in Klein, 1974, p.4).

Although the issue of a new administrative structure for the NHS came to
dominate discussion of NHS policy at Ministerial level for the remainder of the

1960s both the Green Papers on reorganisation in 1968 and 1970 included some mention of the issue of resource allocation. It was increasingly the view that the normative approach to resource allocation was inadequate given the diversity of local circumstances and that a distributional mechanism was required which was independent of the existing supply of resources, so that funds would not automatically be directed to support the existing pattern of services. Those working in less well provided parts of the NHS were increasingly critical of the secrecy and bias of the existing system. Experience was also bringing into question the assumption that progress towards geographical equity could best be achieved through a capital building programme (Klein, 1983, pp. 81-2). At about this time, Richard Crossman, Secretary of State from 1968-1970, was made aware of the importance of the issues of geographical and care group inequalities through a series of scandals in hospitals for the mentally ill and mentally handicapped and from academic research on the persistent inequalities in access to services within the Welfare State (Pollitt, 1984, pp. 51-2). Crossman was disturbed at the amount of capital which was being sucked into London as a result of earlier decisions to expand medical education by extending the existing teaching hospitals rather than building in the provinces. This led to a requirement for increased capacity in central London at the expense of deprived parts of the North. Crossman was put under political pressure from the NHS authorities in the provinces, particularly from the Sheffield RHB, to adopt a fairer system of distribution. Pressure was also brought to bear on Crossman through the Labour Party Social Policy Committee which was worried that "needs" and current allocations were out of step. Crossman's personal advisers and senior officials recommended a population-based formula for resoource allocation. Crossman was sympathetic to this idea, although he recognised that an abrupt shift to a population-based system would be hard on the existing hospitals in the short term. As a result of these discussions of resource allocation the 1970 Labour reorganisation Green Paper included commitment to a new method of resource allocation, so that in the long-run, the basic determinant of the new geographically-based Area Health Authorities' budgets should be:

> '...the population served by the Area, modified to take account of relevant demographic variables, underlying differences in morbidity, the characteristics of the capital plant inherited by each authority, and any special responsibilities undertaken for a wider area and particularly for the special needs of teaching and research.' (DHSS, 1970a, para. 79)

This brief statement embodies all the basic features of the RAWP final report of 1976 and implies a move towards a system of explicit rationing on the basis of resource allocation criteria rather than a normative system based on the attainment of a particular level of service. However, at this stage it was no more than an idea. The mechanics of a future system and its feasibility had not been explored. Its full implementation depended on the establishment of geographical authorities below Regional level, which did not occur until 1974. However, Crossman and his advisers were convinced of the need to begin the process of change within the existing structure. The so-called "Crossman Formula" was the product.

THE CROSSMAN FORMULA, 1971-1975

In 1971/2 a formula based on objective criteria was introduced to guide the distribution of hospital revenue to RHBs. It was to be accompanied by the phasing out of RCCS. The "Crossman Formula" (although it was actually implemented by Sir Keith Joseph) was directly aimed at removing Regional inequalities in the hospital service within a measurable time (ten years). The DHSS was responding to the fact that very little money had been available in the pre-1971 system for redistribution after the demands of RCCS were met and the pace of change had been slow, as the relevant letter to RHB Chairmen made clear:

'At present about two-thirds of the total addition made to hospital revenue each year is pre-empted by new hospitals or other newly completed capital projects. The remaining one-third,..., is available to finance other developments and is distributed by the Department in accordance with the judgement of the relative needs ...But the total money available for distribution is limited, and despite the efforts made over the years to level up standards by giving above-average increments to the Boards considered to be in most need the differences in Regional standards which persist today,...,cannot be justified.'
(DHSS, 1970b, p.1)

In fact as later research was to show, there was little evidence that even the limited capital monies made available under the 1962 Hospital Plan had been spent primarily in areas deprived of capital and revenue (Noyce, Snaith and Trickey, 1974).

In summary, the "Crossman Formula" derived each RHB's 'target' allocation towards which its actual allocations were gradually to move (as in later RAWP), from three elements:

1.   Population - weighted by the national bed occupancy rate for different age and sex groups and adjusted for net patient flows;

2.   Beds - in each speciality weighted by the national average cost per bed per year;

3.   Cases - inpatient, outpatient and day cases weighted by the national average cost per case.

The population factor was given an arbitrary double weight so that the relative contribution to the 'target' of the three elements was population, 0.5, beds, 0.25 and cases, 0.25. A full description of the formula and its method of implementation is given in DHSS (1970b), Griffith (1971) and Maynard and Ludbrook (1980a). The formula was essentially a pragmatic compromise in that independent measures of so-called need were combined with measures of the cost of existing provision (beds) and current activity (cases).

Implicit in the formula (because of the inclusion of the bed factor) was the assumption, present in earlier thinking on resource allocation, that there existed only limited opportunities to substitute the provision of extra revenue (manpower, etc.) for capital deficiencies (beds) (West, 1976, p.88). The bed factor was included to soften the impact of the redistribution on the "over-bedded" RHBs, although the long-term aim was to abandon it. The Secretary of State, Richard Crossman, responsible for introducing the formula, wished to begin the process of redistribution with an approach which did not penalise the existing hospitals too severely. The idea was that the hospital service in "over-provided" parts of the country should be given an opportunity to reduce bed numbers and develop community care and alternatives to hospitalisation before a more radical formula was implemented. Other evidence of caution was the decision that no RHB should actually lose resources but that the under-provided should receive relatively larger increases. As a result, the timescale of implementation was deliberately leisurely. The DHSS did not wish to provoke a political backlash from within the Health Service. At that time, it was thought possible to make progress towards an equitable arrangement relatively painlessly. There was optimism about economic growth, and Richard Crossman is quoted as saying, "I can only equalize on an expanding budget". (Klein, 1983, p.82).

When the Crossman Formula appeared it was generally welcomed for its explicit and formal qualities, and Griffiths (1971) argued that redistribution offered an incentive to RHBs to look critically at their staff and facilities to consider what their 'optimum output' should rationally be. However, he warned that it was a limited, cautious measure which depended for its redistributive success on a growing NHS budget, and was thus in danger of degenerating into a series of piecemeal, marginal adjustments to resource inequalities, dominated by traditional political bargaining rather than rational methods. In the event the implementation of the Formula was severely affected by reductions in the NHS growth rate and was the subject of a number of criticisms.

Gentle and Forsythe (1975) praised the Crossman Formula for being at least "fairer" than its predecessors, since it was based on specified, objective criteria and 50% of the allocation was made independent of existing levels of provision. It overcame the secrecy of the earlier system and its susceptibility to political manipulation; but sub-Regionally very little had changed.

The fullest critical analysis of the Formula was by West (1973) who criticised the population component for making no allowance for the fact that different Regions had different levels of ill-health and need for services. He went on to draw attention to the fact that the case flow and bed stock elements were neither objective measures of need, being based on the size of the Region and its past allocations, nor independent of one another, in that there was a close correlation between the two, since case flow was determined by referral patterns, which were related to existing bed provision. This was in contrast to more optimistic commentators such as Griffiths (1971) who held that the introduction of the Formula would encourage managers to think rationally about priorities and the way resources were used. The argument ran that efficiency improvements could be made while a more equitable distribution was pursued, since Regions with a higher than average provision of beds tended to use them less efficiently than less well endowed Regions. A planned reduction in their resources would stimulate them to use their remaining beds more efficiently. West (1973) argued, by contrast, that the formula could result in possibly excessive incentives to greater efficiency while sacrificing equity. The bed stock and case flow elements in the formula would provide relatively more funds to Regions Regions with higher capacity, thus perpetuating part of the historical variation in Regional standards. In addition, the fact that the case flow element was not fixed but subject to variation caused by decisions in Regions had implications for the attainment of equity. For example, if, in response to a reduction in expenditure, a Region decided to treat fewer cases and maintain its previous style of practice, then the Region's subsequent allocation would fall further because of the case-based element in the Formula. On the other hand, if a Region were able to introduce a lower cost method for treating its cases, it would be able to increase its case flow and in the following period this would increase its revenue. Thus it was not possible with the Crossman Formula, as constituted, to incorporate mechanisms to prevent a change in allocations caused by the behaviour of the hospital authorities themselves. By transferring funds to the more efficient Regions, the cumulative effect of such a process would be to reinforce existing relative advantages and to increase not decrease Regional inequalities (West, 1973; West, 1976; Maynard and Ludbrook, 1980a). There is even anecdotal evidence of hospital authorities artificially inflating their bed numbers for short periods by setting up wards in hospital corridors in order to attract the maximum level of funds through the bed stock element in the Formula!

The Crossman Formula was subject to a range of other criticisms in the literature which are summarised below:

1. The Formula only applied to revenue not capital. There was no attempt to integrate the allocation of capital and revenue. It also only covered hospital services and excluded local authority community health and social services and family practitioner services. However, this was inevitable given the tripartite structure of health services at the time.

2   It needed to be supported by stronger positive discrimination policies to attract medical manpower to less popular parts of the country in line with financial resource shifts (Cooper, 1975, p.71).

3. The Formula did not apply sub-Regionally and there was no formal mechanism for mitigating intra-Regional inequalities. For sub-Regional disparities to be eliminated within the planned ten year period some HMCs (AHAs after 1974) would have had to lose resources, especially in the relatively well-provided Regions, but this was against the principles of the authors of the Formula (Gentle and Forsythe, 1975). It was perhaps not fully appreciated how expensive a "levelling up" policy below Regions would be, given the extent of sub-Regional inequalities. It was calculated in the Oxford Region that to bring all the Areas up to the level of the best for each NHS service in 1974 would cost the equivalent of a 10% increase in the Regional revenue budget plus capital requirements (Rickard, 1974). Gentle and Forsythe (1975) recommended a formula-based approach at all levels in the service for 'fairness' and because it would allow a separation of resource allocation from the use to which resources were to be put by AHAs. This separation was seen as an advantage in giving managers the autonomy to run local services as they saw fit in the light of local needs.

4. The Formula was not genuinely based on health needs between Regions (Bennett and Holland, 1977; Jones and Bourne, 1975). Noyce, Snaith and Trickey (1974) for example, advocated its replacement by a formula modelled on the needs element in the local authority Rate Support Grant (RSG), on the grounds that the RSG had had a more rational and equalising effect on the distribution of local authority resources than the methods used in the NHS (eg, there was a positive correlation between overall local authority expenditure and the proportion of the population in social classes IV and V, but a negative correlation for NHS expenditure). Noyce et al argued that such a formula should be introduced immediately for community services and phased for hospital services. Gentle and Forsythe (1975) proposed a revenue formula based on the population element of the Crossman Formula taking account of the size and age-sex structure of the population, patient flows, teaching, specialised facilities and including an allowance for differential needs of different communities. The authors could see no easy way of assessing needs except to construct an arbitrary index of need from professional and other individuals' value judgements. The size of the allowance to be made for differential need would again have to be arbitrary, though consistently applied.

5. The Crossman Formula sought a fair share-out of financial allocations but there was no related mechanism to ensure that finance was spent in a specified manner and no guarantee that it would lead to the desired distribution of services (West, 1973). The approach was essentially a rationing strategy which made no assumptions about what should result by way of provision. However other writers regarded this as a virtue in an NHS allocation system.

6. The most important deficiency of the Crossman Formula as a redistributive instrument concerned its relationship with the arrangement known as Revenue Consequences of Capital Schemes (RCCS) whereby revenue additions were allocated in response to capital investment (which was in turn planned by criteria having little relation to need). The architects of the Formula planned to phase out RCCS gradually over the first seven years of its implementation, but this proved difficult to accomplish because of the heavy demands on revenue made by capital schemes planned in the 1960s and coming "on stream" in the early 1970s. These schemes had higher running costs than the buildings they replaced. A very high proportion of schemes were associated with the London teaching hospitals. As a result very little growth money was available for redistribution through the Crossman Formula and the impact on territorial inequalities was minimal in the period 1971/2 to 1974/5 when the formula was in operation (Bennett and Holland, 1977). RCCS had the effect of linking revenue quite arbitrarily, in volume and timing, to the extent and timescale of the capital programme, which in turn was the product of past decisions and bore little relationship to population needs.

The Crossman Formula operated throughout the peoriod when Sir Keith Josept was Secretary of State for Social Services (1970-74). Barbara Castle replaced him for Labour in February 1974 and in May 1975, prompted by David Owen, Minister of State for Health, she approved proposals from senior DHSS officials to appoint a Resource Allocation Working Party (RAWP) to look afresh at methods for NHS resource allocation between health authorities. The terms of reference of the Working Party were as follows:

> "To review the arrangements for distributing NHS capital and revenue to RHAs, AHAs and Districts respectively with a view to establishing a method of securing, as soon as practicable, a pattern of distribution responsible objectively, equitably and efficiently to relative need and to make recommendations." (DHSS, 1976c, p.5)

It would appear from this remit that the academic analysis of the Crossman Formula which had taken place in the early 1970s had been influential at least in part. For example a notable commentator on the Crossman Formula had advocated the use of an allocation formula for hospital, GP and local authority health services in 1973:

> '...that removes the remaining influence of historical accidents in past performance and uses instead additional objective measures relating to the needs of each region. The weaknesses of the present formula arise because it is only partially based on the objective needs of the regions through the use of adjusted populations. The other factors depend too heavily on the practices, staff, efficiency and capital of each region to escape the consequences of historical accident.' (West, 1973, p.164).

However academic research into inequalities is most unlikely to have been the principal or even one of the main explanations for the appointment of RAWP in 1976. What other factors contributed to this event?

THE BACKGROUND TO SETTING UP RAWP

Bennett and Holland (1977) who were participants in RAWP admitted soon after, that there was no simple explanation as to why the Working Party was convened at that particular time in 1975. Indeed, there is no systematic and detailed account of the origins of RAWP and the influences on the formation of it policies. However, it is possible to identify from the literature a number of developments which can be linked to its establishment and these will be discussed, in turn. The contribution of research evidence will be considered first, not because it can be rated as an important, direct influence on the decision to set up RAWP in 1975, but more for its contribution to the general climate of opinion about inequalities in resources between different parts of the country. Furthermore, research evidence was a necessary, but by no means sufficient pre-condition for an objective response. It is doubtful if the accumulated research evidence began to exert much influence over thinking on policy until the mid 1970s.

Evidence on Geographical Inequalities in Health and Health Care Resources

For a decade, starting with the work of the economist Feldstein in the early 1960s (Feldstein, 1965 and 1967), social scientists had become increasingly interested in the NHS as a field of study and had been "rediscovering" the regional inequalities in health and health care, particularly within England, which had been all too apparent in the 1930s. By 1975 an impressive body of mainly descriptive research had accumulated. The majority of the work concentrated on inequalities in resources rather than variations in mortality, morbidity, levels of health and the need for health care and the emerging policy debate was similarly focused on equalising resources rather than health outcomes.

Although there was evidence that since 1948 there had been some reduction in spatial inequalities in resources (Hollingsworth, 1981) major disparities remained. There were also disturbing accounts of discrepancies in quality of care between the acute and long-stay sectors. Although it could not automatically be assumed that because an authority had below average provision it should get more, the extent of variation was so great that redistributive policy implications were probably unavoidable (Buxton and Klein, 1975).

1. Revenue and Capital Resources at Regional Level

A series of research studies in the 1960s and early 1970s by health economists at Exeter and later at York Universities documented the continuing unequal distribution of hospital beds and other resources. Cooper and Culyer used 31 indices derived from official sources, including data on expenditure, beds, manpower and physical facilities for each of the 15 RHBs to chart the extent of inequalities in acute services (Cooper and Culyer, 1970; 1971; 1972; Cooper, 1975, pp.63 - 67). Consistently high levels of provision were recorded in the Metropolitan RHBs and Liverpool, and consistently low levels in East Anglia and Sheffield. Parallel work at York by Maynard demonstrated a similar Regional pattern of inequalities in provision and expenditure for hospital psychiatric services (Maynard, 1972; Maynard and Tingle, 1976). Evidence of inequalities in provision was also gathered beyond the hospital service. Noyce, Snaith and Trickey (1974) calculated the distribution of expenditure per capita for 1971/2 at Regional level for family doctor, local authority community health and NHS hospital services. The authors found considerable inequalities in expenditure in all three sectors, but to their surprise, dispersion about the mean was greatest for hospital services which were nominally under central control and least for local authority services. Regional hospital expenditure as a proportion of the national mean varied between +41% and -23%.u

These studies combined to suggest that provision might indeed be inversely related to need as Hart had claimed when he coined the term 'Inverse Care Law' on the strength of an interpretation of earlier, cruder data (Hart, 1971). Hart's work was substantiated to some extent by further analyses. Jones and Bourne (1976) used a range of simple indicators of need and provision at county level for 1971, covering hospital, GP and local authority social services to show that provision and need were poorly matched. West and Lowe (1976) studied routine indices of need, provision and use of the child health services at Regional level and concluded that they were badly matched.

There were also close correlations between the various health care supply variables studied. There was no evidence of a resource deficiency in one aspect of provision being compensated for by good provision in another (eg capital for revenue and vice versa). Hospital expenditure at Regional level was found in one study to be positively correlated with expenditure on GP and local authority health services and with the proportion of the population in the higher socio-economic groups. In addition hospital capital and revenue expenditure levels were positively correlated (Noyce, Snaith and Trickey, 1974). Furthermore, there was no evidence to presume that Regions with low endowments of manpower, capital or expenditure had higher quality inputs. The better endowed areas tended, for example, to attract better qualified staff (Lavers and Rees, 1972).

Such work raised a number of questions about the reasons for the existence of such disparities and whether they could be justified or not. The sheer extent of differences in provision raised questions about the rationality and principles behind previous resource allocation methods. For example, Cooper (1975) argued that access to teaching hospitals as "centres of excellence" should be roughly equal to all, irrespective of Region. Yet in the 1960s he showed that while Wessex RHB had no teaching beds at all, the North West Metropolitan RHB had one teaching bed for every 615 people!

These data on inequalities in provision had profound implications since they implied inequalities in access and utilisation, although in the main, these aspects were not studied in such depth. It had been shown in earlier economic analyses that the supply of health care resources sustained its own demand and thereby created unequal utilisation rates. Feldstein had demonstrated that Regions with more beds hospitalised more people and for longer than Regions with fewer beds (Feldstein, 1965; 1967). Logan and colleagues (1972) went on to show that in Mersey RHB which had one of the highest bed:population ratios, the extra bed availability led to the admission of less severe cases for longer hospital stays. Recent research indicates that this relationship between resource levels and activity rates still holds. For example, a study of age and sex standardised rates for common surgical operations by RHA found that 'excess' levels of hospital funding as defined by RAWP were strongly related to higher rates for surgery (McPherson, Strong, Epstein and Jones, 1981). The implication of research in the 1960s seemed to be that the high numbers of beds per capita such as in the Metropolitan RHB could not be justified in terms of conventional indices of medical and social need, particularly when the level of provision in the poorly endowed Regions was compared. As a result, it was agreed by some commentators that there was scope for reducing the number of acute beds in the well-endowed Regions, redistributing the resources elsewhere and still continuing to treat the same number of patients. This could be done if throughput were raised to the national average, thus making an efficiency gain through a more equitable distribution (Griffiths, 1971). It was even possible to justify a reduction in the number of patients treated in the better-off Regions since there was little evidence that their higher admission rates were sickness-related. It was plausible for economists to argue that some of the people receiving treatment in the well-off Regions had less need of it than people waiting to be treated in poorly endowed Regions (Ludbrook and Maynard, 1983, p.233).

2. Inequalities at Sub-Regional Level

Choosing the most appropriate level of aggregation is a particularly important decision in studies of spatial inequalities since it may well alter the results of the analysis. The geographical comparisons of health care and welfare resources made in the 1960s took place largely at Regional level because of the limited availability of more local data, particularly in the NHS, where the RHB was the lowest geographically-based management tier before 1974. However, commonsense hinted that variations sub-Regionally might be even greater than at Regional level. The Area profiles prepared by DHSS in 1973 as part of the preparation for reorganisation in 1974 provided an excellent opportunity to study the distribution of resources within Regions. The general conclusion was that variations between the new AHAs were much greater than between the new RHAs. Klein and Buxton (1974) used data on NHS revenue expenditure for 1971/72 and applied it to the new RHA and AHA populations. They discovered that while the Regional range varied from +41% to -23% about the national average, the AHAs within the Trent Region for example, ranged from +34% in Sheffield to -62% in Rotherham. In the West Midlands, the range was from +20% in Solihull to -69% in Sandwell. The Areas with the most resources were those with teaching hospitals providing some Regional services. The researchers were well aware of the importance of patient flows and the effect of specialised services in particular centres in interpreting these results, but concluded that even allowing for flows, it was still difficult to account in full for many of the variations. However, they did not discuss the extent to which their results might, in part, at least , be explicable in terms of variations in treatment costs and case-mix between different sorts of hospitals. As in other studies, it was found that Areas with low levels of hospital resources tended (although there were exceptions) to be poor in other local authority health services, but that the geographical variations in the level of local authority services were less marked, partly as a result of the fact that local authority administrative boundaries represented genuine boundaries to patient movement. One of the worst examples of multiple NHS and local authority "under-provision" given by Klein and Buxton (1974) was Walsall which was 50% below the Regional average for hospital revenue, 17% below average on local authority health services and 42% below average on Executive Council (GP, dental, pharmaceutical and ophthalmic services) expenditure. Further more detailed analysis of the distribution of beds and revenue per capita between different specialties cast doubt on whether some AHAs were capable of providing a 'comprehensive service' even in the basic acute specialities as envisaged under the 1974 reorganisation plans (Buxton and Klein, 1975). Variations in beds and expenditure per capita were as great in the basic acute specialties in which it would have been reasonable to expect AHAs to be fairly self-sufficient (eg general medicine, general surgery, maternity, etc.), as in the more rarified specialties.

It was recognised that hospital catchments rather than administrative areas would have been more relevant when considering disparities in acute services, but Buxton and Klein made the important point that judgements would still have to be made about the desirability of maintaining the existing pattern of flows, since some might represent flows of 'convenience' and be 'rational' and others might be the product of 'necessity' and result from difficulty of access. They also warned against the temptation to draw facile policy conclusions from their data. With a DHSS policy at the time to reduce the number of acute beds per capita, they warned that AHAs with less than average provision were not necessarily under-provided. They admitted however, that usable criteria for deciding an appropriate level of provision such as morbidity levels, were not self-evidently available, other than simply population size. (Buxton and Klein, 1975, p. 348). This was the task RAWP faced.

Interest in issues of sub-Regional equity was further fuelled by other studies at AHA level, which came to conclusions similar to those reported above, namely that:

1. sub-Regional variation over a wide range of NHS and local authority services was far greater than inter-Regional variation in resources;

2.   there was less geographical variation in levels of provision of local authority services than NHS services;

3.   there was no evidence of expenditure in one sector compensating for deficiencies in another (Jones and Masterman, 1976; Rickard, 1976).

Studies began to include increasingly sophisticated adjustments to allow for factors such as cross-boundary flows, teaching costs and Regional specialties in the relative expenditure of different AHAs so that fair comparisons could be made (Rickard, 1976). Even after controlling as far as possible for such factors, Rickard showed that out of 90 AHAs, 49 were within £3 of the national average expenditure per capita of general hospital, but 22 AHAs had expenditure more than £3 under the national average and 19 AHAs had expenditure more than £3 greater than the national average. Since Rickard's work was carried out on behalf of DHSS officials responsible for setting up RAWP and since he was a DHSS member of two of its Sub-Groups on Revenue and Capital Allocations it is not surprising that adjustments similar to those reported in Rickard (1976) were included in the RAWP formula.

A general point about the studies above is the fact that most but not all comparisons tended to be made between often arbitrarily-defined administrative units rather than between areas with characteristics relevant to health service accessibility, use and need. This was no doubt largely because of the availability of data by administrative areas. In the process, a number of dimensions of inequality which have subsequently received attention were not fully addressed, particularly the health service problems of socially deprived inner city districts and the rural-urban split in health care provision. The rural dimension has been consistently ignored in policy terms. Heller (1979), for example, argued that NHS provision in rural England as a whole was inadequate with highly restricted access to services for the majority of the population due to problems of transport, shortage of services, the movement to centralised provision and poor quality provision. Evidence from East Anglia showed that those who had greatest "need" for health services (as revealed through utilisation rates) especially the elderly and women with children, had the most problems in getting to services and that all the rural Districts in East Anglia had levels of NHS expenditure well below the national average. However, East Anglia was characterised by relatively low infant and maternal mortality and low overall mortality rates.

3. Manpower Inequalities

Although a number of the above studies on health care resource inequalities included data on health manpower inequalities, most were focused on indicators such as beds, revenue and capital, for which data were more plentiful. However, the distribution of professional manpower would seem to be equally, if not more important in certain respects. No attempt will be made to draw together all the evidence on manpower inequalities which was available in the late 1960s and 1970s, but merely to indicate the main features of the situation. Looking at hospital doctors, Cooper and Culyer (1972) indicated that additions to the stock of doctors since 1948 had served to reinforce the pre-existing unequal distribution. There had been no central direction and no effective inducements had been offered to influence staff to more unattractive areas or specialties. The Central Medical Manpower Committee at the Ministry of Health operated on the basis of professional, as opposed to population needs, criteria in allocating consultant appointments by hospital and by specialty. There were massive variations in consultant, registrar and junior manpower. For example, in the early 1970s, Newcastle had twice as many gynaecologists per female as Sheffield. Griffiths (1971) reported a similar picture with inequalities closely related in the main to levels of bed provision. On the GP side, despite policies stretching back to 1948 to try to ensure an 'adequate' number of general practitioners in each area of the country (Butler, Bevan and Taylor, 1973), the BMA Planning Unit was still concerned in 1970 at the maldistribution of GPs and variations in list sizes by Region (Knox, 1979). Although the proportion of GPs working in 'designated' areas (i.e where the average list-size was over 2,500 patients) had fallen from 44% of GPs in 1952 to less than 18% in 1961 (Cooper, 1975) and only 13% in 1977 (it actually increased in the period 1963-71), there was still a strong Regional bias. In the 1970s, average list sizes were still significantly higher in the North than the South (Maynard and Ludbrook, 1982, p. 103), and in deprived rather than affluent parts of the country, lending some support to the idea of an 'inverse care law' for family doctor services (Knox, 1979). In fact, the data showing improvements in list sizes (eg. Butler, Bevan and Taylor, 1973) may have given too favourable a picture of the distribution since no account was taken of the relative needs/demands of the populations served (Buxton and Klein, 1979).

4. Geographical Variation in Mortality

As well as evidence on per capita differences in the availability of resources of all kinds, what evidence was available about the needs of populations? Morbidity data were scanty, but evidence of geographical differences in mortality had been collected for many years and was well-known. The literature on the subject is extensive and no attempt will be made to do justice to it (eg. Howe, 1963; Gardner, Winter and Barker, 1984; Charlton, Hartley, Silver and Holland, 1983). In brief, the NHS inherited marked Regional differences in mortality. For example, in 1949 the all-causes standardised mortality ratio (SMR) for Durham and Northumberland was 113; that for Greater London, 93; and the SMR for the remainder of the South East, 90. In 1978, the pattern was similar (Maynard and Ludbrook, 1982, p. 102). More specifically, a number of studies documented marked spatial variations in infant mortality (often regarded as a good proxy for the overall health status of a population) even in the 1970s and indicated that its distribution mirrored the quality of life, with lowest levels in the affluent towns and suburbs of South East England (Ashford, Read and Riley, 1973; Coates and Rawstron, 1971; DHSS, 1980a). Variation appeared to be controlled largely by spatial variations in socio-economic factors such as class and income structure, though it was also influenced by the quality of health care available, which in turn, seemed to be better in more affluent areas (Knox, 1981).

5. Trends in Inequality of Resources and Needs

In absolute terms, the supply of health service resources had increased in all Regions since the inception of the NHS. In relative terms, the evidence suggested that inequalities in financial resources, manpower and buildings were virtually untouched in the period 1948-62 with the possibility that they may even have widened in certain respects (Cooper and Culyer, 1972, p.52). In the period 1962-1967, Cooper adduced evidence that inequalities appeared to be increasing, particularly in medical manpower (Cooper, 1975, p.64). However, taking the period since the beginning of the NHS to 1971/72, he showed that inequalities in revenue per capita had improved such that the revenue of the poorest RHBs equalled a higher proportion of the revenue of the best-off RHBs by the end of the period. Abel-Smith (1978, p.22) cites similar data produced by DHSS for the House of Commons Expenditure sub-Committee on Social Services, in which revenue allocations per capita to RHBs varied less widely in 1971/72 than in 1950/51. In 1971/72 the best off Region received about a third more than the Region with the lowest allocation. In 1950/51 the best provided Region had received over twice the allocation per head of the worst provided Region. On the other hand the rankings were little changed. Sheffield RHB had had the smallest revenue and bed allocation in 1948 with 9.1 beds per 1000 population, as against the highest, South West Metropolitan RHB, with 14.8 beds per 1000.

In 1976 South West Thames RHA still had the highest bed allocation and only Oxford RHA had fewer beds per capita than Trent RHA (formerly Sheffield RHB) (Maynard and Ludbrook, 1980b, p.38). In terms of spatial mortality variation, the general trend was towards a narrowing of differentials over the period since 1948 (Hollingsworth, 1981, pp.274-5), although inequalities were remarkably persistent (Maynard and Ludbrook, 1982, p.102). This narrowing was not a uniform effect. Knox (1981) studied the relative change in infant mortality by local authority areas for 1949-52 and 1970-72 and showed that the overall intensity of spatial inequality had changed very little, though the relative position of some areas had changed.

6. Inequalities in Health Service Resources Between Constituent Parts of the U.K.

By comparison with studies of Regional inequalities in England, little if any, attention was given in research in the 1960s and 1970s to the existence of inequalities in resources between the countries of the U.K. Given that the National Health Service covers the whole of the U.K., it may at first sight seem surprising that this was so. On crude measures of inequality there had been significant differences for many years. However, it was not until Maynard and Ludbrook published a series of papers after RAWP and its Scottish, Welsh and Northern Ireland equivalents had already been implemented, that these inequalities were quantified (Maynard and Ludbrook, 1980a; 1980b; 1980c). Despite the fact that expenditure per capita in the four Thames Regions was higher than the rest of England and Wales, it fell short of expenditure in Scotland and Northern Ireland (Hunter, 1983, pp.59-62). In 1975 there were on average 114.3 doctors per 100,000 population in the U.K., but 93.5 doctors per 100,000 population in Trent Region, 114.1 in Wales, 146.5 in North West Thames and 160.3 in Scotland (Maynard and Ludbrook, 1980c). The Royal Commission on the National Health Service noted that Scotland had 50% more hospital doctors and 40% more nurses per capita than England and Wales (Royal Commission on the NHS, 1979, p.26). In 1976 the U.K. bedstock per 1000 population was 100, while England had 95 beds per 1000, Wales 100, Northern Ireland 128 and Scotland, 132. Calculations of the overall NHS budgets in the different countries in the late 1970s indicated that Scotland's per capita budget was 20% higher than the rest of the U.K. and Northern Ireland's still higher. The same authors revealed that the overall growth of expenditure had been faster in Scotland and Northern Ireland than in England and Wales (Gray and Mooney, 1981, p.5). Gray and Mooney also rejected on empirical grounds the claim that the higher level of funding was justified in Scotland because of higher mortality and morbidity (Gray and Mooney, 1981).

How did these differences in funding come about and why have they been so little debated? When the NHS started, Scotland was relatively better provided compared to England but facilities in Wales were as bad or worse than the bad parts of England. In the early days of the NHS, hospital development in South Wales and North West Wales was given a high priority and by the 1960s per capita expenditure in Wales far exceeded England, and Scotland had enhanced its relative position still further (Godber, 1975). Godber explained the relative success of Wales, Scotland and Northern Ireland in securing resources in the 1940s, 1950s and 1960s in political terms, through their independent advocacy for funds for health service development over the heads of the English Regions which lacked the necessary representation as distinct, political entities. The most successful canvassing was by the Scots who have had a Minister in the Cabinet since 1948. On the other hand, the Welsh Office was created as late as 1964, yet even before this, Wales had benefited disproportionately from increases in NHS funding (Hunter, 1983, p.63).

The answer to the second question as to why the discussion of reform of the inequalities between different parts of the U.K. had been muted despite the attention given to inequalities within countries, is not spelled out in the literature. However, it is clear that there is considerable political resistance to the idea of UK-wide redistribution, in the form of arguments about decentralisation and in favour of national identity. On a bureaucratic level there are practical obstacles in the form of the separate administrative structures of the NHS in the four countries. In the early to mid-1970s when devolution was a live political issue the political pressures were even more strongly against introducing a UK system of resource allocation (Maynard and Ludbrook, 1983).

7. Accounting for the Persistence of Geographical Inequalities in Provision

It is not possible in this space to develop a coherent account of how and why geographical inequalities in provision and utilisation persisted despite the advent of the NHS, since the issue is too wide-ranging. However, a range of overlapping explanations are hinted at in the literature on political, economic, organisational and technical levels and are worth a brief outline if only because they prefigure some of the reasons put forward subsequently to account for the constraints on the implementation of the RAWP approach. The main sorts of explanations can be summarised as follows:

a. A major characteristic of NHS planning up to the mid-1970s had been its relative weakness in the face of powerful vested interests which had tended to be influential in decision-making. Acute hospital consultants dominated the process of defining health need (Ham, 1981). The fragmentation of the NHS structure into three parts before 1974 made comprehensive planning and authoritative management impossible (Griffiths, 1971). Furthermore the fact that the teaching hospitals were able to negotiate for funds directly with the Ministry of Health had led to their receiving preferential treatment, thus perpetuating inequalities in provision. For example, the 1962 Hospital Plan had the supposed aim of building district general hospitals in parts of the country which lacked them, yet one of its major results was a series of rebuilding schemes at London teaching hospitals (Bennett and Holland, 1977). The London teaching hospitals had influential supporters in the House of Lords and were able to augment the generosity of government with their own trust funds! In addition, they were able to profit from the government decision in the early 1960s to expand medical education at the existing teaching centres on the grounds that this would be cheaper than building anew in the provinces. As a result London teaching hospitals were able to obtain resources for expansion.

b. Methods of allocation of financial resources based on historical patterns of funding left very little scope for redistribution (Griffiths, 1971). The Ministry of Health had at its disposal only relatively small sums of money which were not already spoken for. The one potentially powerful redistributive tool open to the Ministry of Health was its control over major capital building. Yet the meagre level of capital investment rendered this ineffective, since funds tended to be devoted to the upkeep of existing hospitals rather than provision of new facilities in poor RHBs (Godber, 1975).

c. In the period before 1974, because of RCCS, the NHS lacked sufficient uncommitted resources for redistribution which would have enabled "levelling up" to take place (ie bringing the poorest Region up to the level of funding of the richest without halting expenditure growth in the richest Region). However politicians and administrators were generally

reluctant to see the better-off areas of the country either halted or
losing resources in a redistributive process. Godber argued for levelling
up in England on the basis that:

> 'Because health services develop even locally in an almost organic way,
> it is really not possible - even if it were desirable - suddenly to cut
> short what is available in one area and give it elsewhere. If this
> happens the degree of frustration amongst those concerned would be such
> as would certainly bring forth justified and loud protest.'
> (Godber, 1975, p.72)

For politicians, the cause of their reluctance was even clearer. Enoch
Powell, for instance, reflecting on his time as Minister of Health, noted
the 'political odium of being seen to reduce expenditure' (quoted in
Cooper, 1975). Before Richard Crossman's period as Secretary of State for
Health and Social Services (1968-70) it is difficult to detect the
political will to tackle geographical inequalities in the availability of
hospital resources.

d.   Redistribution through the "levelling up" of resources between RHBs which
was the least contentious option would have been very expensive (Buxton and
Klein, 1975). Rickard calculated in 1974 prices that it would cost £5
million per year in Oxford RHA to bring all the AHAs in the Region up to
the level of service of the best provided AHA (cited in Klein, 1975, p.
98). Redistribution away from the richest Regions would have been cheaper
and quicker but had high "frictional costs", in the form of political
opposition and controversy. However, a third option, the selective
distribution of growth monies to the least well endowed Regions while the
remainder stood still, although lowering the resistance of the
over-provided Regions, would have meant a long-drawn-out process,
unattractive to politicians eager for results. Whichever method of
Regional redistribution was contemplated, the timespan for implementation
would be measured in years rather than months. The major disparities,
however, were at AHA and District level where services were delivered. To
deal with these differences so that populations at AHA level would have
equal opportunity of access to health services, would take even longer; far
beyond the time horizons of most Ministers. This did not necessarily mean
equalising the level of services provided by each AHA, since patients would
continue to flow across administrative boundaries for treatment. Richard
Crossman identified Regional resource inequalities as an important policy
problem while Secretary of State for Health and Social Services. His
conclusion, faced with these dilemmas, was that there was no easy way to
aid the 'underprivileged areas with a major legitimate grievance' without
some cut-backs in the better-off areas (Crossman, 1977).

e.   Redistribution involving sacrifices by certain Regions so that other
Regions could attain parity might have been facilitated had there been an
accepted and consistent conception of a desirable level of health services
for each locality. The norms used in planning had varied over the years
and there was a lack of data on the factors which influenced the use and
need for health resources in different parts of the country (Ford, 1972).
Commentators bemoaned the absence of a system for measuring the need for
health services. Even after the introduction of the Crossman Formula the
Labour Under-Secretary of State for Health stated in 1972:

> 'We had not developed any acceptable system of measuring the relative
> needs of regions.'

A year later he said:

> '..at present we have neither a comprehensive assessment of need nor a thorough going audit, as it were, of existing stock.' (quoted in Cooper, 1975, p. 70)

f. There were also doubts about the administrative feasibility of redistributing physical and manpower resources as opposed to funds. Klein argued that such resources:

> '....cannot be switched by administrative fiat from one geographical area to another. Beds cannot be switched from one hospital to another; neither can consultants. There is limited scope for transferring registrar posts from one area to another...The problem is compounded by the fact that many of the deprived areas are socially unattractive; providing extra resources to improve the facilities will not necessarily guarantee the skilled manpower required... As the experience of general practice has shown, offering financial incentives to persuade doctors to move into areas of shortage does not necessarily work' (Klein, 1975, p. 99)

g. Inequalities in the distribution of resources in relation to population were exacerbated by secular shifts in population out of the central core of the major cities and into the periphery. The major teaching hospitals and centres of health service activity were located mainly in the inner city areas of declining population.

Despite the problems which any redistributive mechanism would encounter, the accumulated evidence had clearly demonstrated the inequalities and irrationality of the prevailing distribution of resources between the NHS Regions. Although concepts such as "need" for, or "adequacy" of health services were understandably vague, commentators increasingly implied that a more rational and fairer system for the allocation of NHS financial resources could and should be introduced. For instance, having reviewed the evidence of inequality in resource availability, Michael Cooper concluded that:

> In the absence,...of any reliable or accepted indicator of need, per capita equality would appear a more rational goal than the perpetuation of historical chance.' (Cooper, 1975, p.67)

The 1974 Reorganisation

The weight of evidence on geographical inequality and on the weaknesses in the Crossman formula was reflected in the explicit commitment in the 1974 reorganisation White Paper to deal with the historical inequalities in the distribution of resources in the NHS:

> 'The allocations of available funds to health authorities will be designed progressively to reduce the disparities between the resources available to different regions, and to achieve standards and improvements in services with due regard to national, regional and area priorities. The new information systems and other methods of assessment and review of services should help to ensure that the bases used for allocating funds meet these objectives with increasing effectiveness.' (DHSS, 1972b, p. 40, para. 160)

It is probably true to say that the main impetus to the setting up of RAWP in 1975 lies in the events and objectives of the 1974 reorganisation (Bennett and Holland, 1977). The reorganisation itself created for the first time an administrative tier (AHA) with statutory responsibility for service delivery to a specific geographical population, unlike the former HMCs. Resource distribution became an issue of increased significance. The development of AHAs enabled meaningful comparisons to be drawn between the endowments of different administrative units for the first time. In 1973, as part of the preparation for reorganisation each 'shadow' AHA was asked to prepare an Area profile setting out the level of provision of hospital resources, GP services and local authority community health services within its boundaries. Data from these profiles showed more clearly than ever before the extent of variations at local level and were used in a number of influential studies (eg. Klein and Buxton, 1974; Buxton and Klein, 1975)

The new AHAs not only meant that the lowest tier of the NHS was geographically based for the first time, but also that AHA members came to identify with the needs of the communities within their boundaries. AHAs proved more powerful politically than their predecessors, the Hospital Management Committees (HMCs) and were quickly alert to any deficiencies in the resources at their disposal compared with more fortunate parts of the Service. As authorities in their own right they were in a position to criticise the sub-Regional allocation of funds.

Not only was the AHA to be geographically based, but it was established as an effective, self-governing, planning unit responsible for providing '... comprehensive health services designed to meet the needs of the communities within its districts' (DHSS, 1972b p.10, para. 42). A responsibility to plan for 'communities' within the Area was difficult to discharge in situations where an AHA was dependent on other, better provided, AHAs for the provision of essential services to patients living within its administrative boundaries. In these cases, pressure for redistribution was generated on the grounds of self-sufficiency. Yet the reorganisation White Paper also envisaged collaboration between AHAs in these circumstances:

'There will be many instances in which one AHA will provide services for another and AHAs generally will collaborate with each other in matters of common interest..., some AHAs may need to arrange for certain services to be provided from neighbouring areas. In some instances, the area authorities concerned will be situated in different regions, which will mean collaboration across regional boundaries.
(DHSS, 1972b, p.11, para. 50)

There thus appears to have been some ambiguity in the guidance issued for the 1974 reorganisation as to the relative importance AHAs should attach on the one hand to providing a comprehensive range of services for their residents and on the other, to ensuring access to health care for residents wherever it might be available.

The 1974 reorganisation contributed to the establishment of RAWP more directly since it was generally seen by the DHSS as an opportunity to improve a wide range of NHS management functions including resource allocation and planning. A new planning system which was to be explicitly needs-based was proposed and it was logical therefore to expect that the resource allocation process should also similarly respond to health need. Among the criticisms of the Crossman Formula made at that time was the view that it was insufficiently responsive to diffential need for health care between different Regions (Noyce, Snaith and Trickey, 1974; Jones and Bourne, 1975). By contrast to resource allocation procedures in the NHS, commentators pointed to the local authority Rate Support Grant as an example of a needs-based approach to resource allocation which had resulted in a seemingly more rational distribution of levels of local authority expenditure in relation to the needs of areas than obtained in the NHS. According to Bennett and Holland (1977) the desire to make a transition from 'muddling through' or 'disjointed incrementalism' to 'rational planning' (in

which objectives are established and the best means of achieving them
identified) lay at the heart of the 1974 reorganisation and accounted for the
attraction felt at the time for an approach to resource allocation responsive to
relative need. The authors (both of whom were directly involved in RAWP) saw a
more rational approach as worth aiming for, despite its many practical problems
(eg. inadequate data, unknown inter-dependencies between facts and values,
etc.) and, in the spirit of RAWP, backed the use of what data were available and
proxy measures of need as a basis for reallocation of resources, rather than no
system at all.

Establishment of DHSS Regional Group

In 1972 the DHSS had set up a Regional Group with responsibility for developing
and maintaining contact with health authorities. For the first time, there was
a Division (later two) within the Regional Group with specific, geographically
determined Regional liaison functions. The establishment of the Regional Group
was clearly linked to the objective in the 1974 reorganisation to organise and
plan health services on a geographical basis in relation to population needs.
This meant bringing together assessments of need based not only on client
groups, but also on geographical units. It was thus logical that the Regional
Group should take an interest in geographical resource allocation. Unlike the
Divisions in the Services Development Group, with their focus on a particular
service or care group, the Regional Group was able to take a broad overview of
the planning and resource allocation requirements of Regions. Officials in the
Regional Division with responsibility for liaison with RHAs commissioned
analyses of resource distribution (eg. Rickard, 1974). The scale of inequality
offended their sense of logic and administrative consistency. Furthermore their
desire for change was supported by the recommendations of a DHSS devolution
working party which had been set up around the time of the 1974 reorganisation
to consider the respective roles, levels of autonomy and lines of accountability
between DHSS and the two new tiers of health authorities. The devolution
working party urged a change in resource allocation methods as crucial to
effective devolution to the new authorities in line with the objectives of
reorganisation.

A characteristic feature of the Regional Group's style in the later 1970s was to
set up joint DHSS-NHS committees as a way of influencing and ensuring the
cooperation of the NHS in policy initiatives. Two such were the Resource
Allocation Working Party and the London Health Planning Consortium. The Group
believed that the recommendations which emerged from joint DHSS-NHS working
parties would carry greater weight with the Health Service than proposals
produced by civil servants in isolation. The Regional Group was increasingly
concerned to avoid the criticism from the NHS that it was interfering
unnecessarily in NHS activities. Thus it had to devise a means of incorporating
senior NHS officials in joint policy developments. The membership of the
Resource Allocation Working Party was carefully constructed to include roughly
equal representation of DHSS officials and a range of NHS managers from
different disciplines and parts of the country, together with an academic
epidemiologist who became a member of all three of the Working Party's
sub-groups. The chairman and secretariat were from DHSS. The purpose of these
arrangements was to increase commitment throughout the NHS to the Working
Party's proposals, while at the same time keeping Departmental control over the
general direction of the recommendations (Butts, Irving and Whitt, 1981, p.33).
However, there were no clinicians on the Working Party which severely reduced
the credibility of its recommendations in the eyes of the medical profession,
particularly hospital doctors.

Development of Social Indicators

One of the main weaknesses of the Crossman Formula as a redistributive mechanism for upsetting the historical distribution of services, was its reliance in part on variables reflecting the supply of health service resources (cases and beds) rather than data on health care need. In order to improve on the existing formula some means of measuring the relative need for health care of a Region was required in order to ascertain the share of available revenue to which each Region was entitled. Since the mid-1960s the "social indicator movement" had been developing a variety of socio-economic indicators of well-being and "quality of life", primarily to assist government and public bodies in their decision-making (Shonfield and Shaw, 1972). The rise of the "social indicator movement" was to a great extent based on the belief that the provision of information in areas previously neglected would result in better, more rational government decisions, based more on fact and social reality and less on hidden subjective judgements (Carley, 1981, pp. 87-111). One of the most significant methodological developments in the UK was the production of statistical indicators of territorial need useful for identifying geographical areas or population sub-groups towards which policy might be directed (see Carley, 1981, for a detailed account). By the early 1970s policy-makers were becoming familiar with the potential value of using indicators of need to guide resource allocation and social scientists in turn were developing the necessary techniques to enable indicators to be used routinely. In the 1970s territorial indicators came to be used by government for three purposes: to distinguish public authorities to be given special assistance because of the unusual concentration of social problems they faced; to provide a basis for allocating general grants to local and health authorities; and to help local authorities give priority to certain districts within their boundaries (Glennerster, 1981).

Work specifically on the subject of the need for health care, territorial justice and the spatial distribution of welfare resources and expenditure was beginning to accumulate from the late 1960s. For example, Bleddyn Davies' study of inequalities in the distribution of local authority social services' provision was the first in Britain to develop indices of comparative need (Davies, 1968). In the USA, Health Status Indexes were being designed to measure the comparative need for health care of geographical areas using either mortality or morbidity data or based on proxy measures of need such as the demographic structure and social class composition of populations associated with particular levels of health (for example, Berg, 1973).

Jones and Bourne (1976) identified a range of territorial "need" indicators based on routine data, of a type which were notably absent from the Crossman Formula and suggested that similar indicators could be used in a developed form in a modified NHS resource allocation mechanism. The authors reviewed routinely available sources of data and fixed on the following possible indicators of "need" and the adequacy of provision: crude mortality rates, sickness absence days, the change in SMR, 1969-1972, available geriatric beds per 1000 population over 65 years, available obstetric beds per 1000 females 15-44 years, available beds in the other non-psychiatric specialties per 1000 population, percent of GP lists with fewer than 2,500 patients, occupants of Part III homes per 1,000 population over 65 years and occupants of local authority children's homes per 1000 population under 18 years. Although such studies may seem crude, they demonstrate the influence which the "social indicators movement" was exerting on public policy-makers at the time. For example, while Jones and Bourne (1976) were aware of the problems of defining criteria against which the current distribution of resources could be judged, as well as the difficulties of quantifying differences and obtaining the necessary data, they were nonetheless sure that resource allocation based on measures of "need", however imperfectly constructed, would result in a fairer, more rational outcome.

Howard Glennerster sums up the considerable significance of the "social indicators movement" for the inception of RAWP as follows:

'The failure to achieve any significant narrowing of geographical inequalities in access to hospital care especially, may be variously laid at the door of entrenched medical interests and the sheer inertia of incremental budgeting practices. [However] even with the political will to change this situation little might have happened without the technical means of quantifying the extent to which resources would have to be redeployed in order to make equal access a reality.'
(Glennerster, 1981, p.40)

Role of the British Medical Association

Although the London teaching hospitals and their consultants had profited from the pre-1970 resource allocation system, resentment against them was building up, not only in the RHBs and their successor RHAs and AHAs, but also within the medical profession itself. Antagonism between London and the provinces led provincial doctors who felt deprived, to press for the introduction of a redistributive mechanism of resource allocation. The Council of the British Medical Association (BMA) played an influential part behind the scenes in pushing for RAWP. However, the BMA was distinctly less enthusiastic about redistribution when the RAWP proposals were published and the NHS budget was entering a period of reduced growth (Anonymous, 1976b)

Prospects for Public Spending

The establishment of the Resource Allocation Working Party and innovations in the techniques of quantifying territorial inequalities and allocating resources have also been linked to the deteriorating economic climate of the mid-1970s and the need therefore, for systems, of rationing resources. However, in 1975 when the Working Party was established, there was little appreciation within DHSS or the NHS of the extent to which expectations of growth would have to change. Yet by the time RAWP reported in 1976, it was apparent that in future, NHS expenditure growth would be strictly limited and lower than it had been in preceding years. It was argued by the British Medical Journal at a relatively early stage that with less money to go round, it was more important than before to ensure that it was distributed in an equitable way (Anonymous, 1975a). In addition, the Crossman Formula had been designed to allow the budgets of the worst-off Regions to increase at a faster rate than those of the best-off ones, the success of which depended on an overall increase in NHS resources. The Crossman approach had not been formulated to produce reallocation on reduced or no growth. Faced with stringency it is unsurprising that attention should focus on developing new techniques for rationing the available resources and that such techniques should be required to be "objective" and "rational" so that political opposition could be minimised. However, it would be a mistake to see the setting up of the Working Party as a direct response to perceived economic change. Its roots predate the economic shocks of 1975/76. However, economic conditions have played an important part in RAWP's implementation since 1976. David Owen summarised the significance of economic conditions for RAWP as follows:

'It is perhaps a practical fact of life that the problems of redistribution can only be faced at a time of economic difficulty, even though, theoretically, it must be easier to redress inequalities at a time of economic growth.' (Owen, 1976, p. 49)

Subsequent events have shown how difficult geographical redistribution becomes when instead of being based on differential growth, it involved reductions in resources in certain areas to benefit others.

Political Will

Between 1968 and 1970, Richard Crossman put Regional inequalities in health care back onto the health policy agenda after nearly 20 years of relative neglect. His period in office as Secretary of State at the DHSS coincided with the rediscovery of inequality despite the existence of the Welfare State, by academic social policy analysts with whom he was in particularly close contact. Crossman was made forcibly aware of inequalities between geographical areas and between care groups. He was made aware that during a period of rapid growth in health expenditure, spatial inequalities of resources had actually widened. The The Hospital and Health Services Review was clear in its view that:

> 'If anyone is to be given blame or credit [for RAWP] it should be whoever put it to Richard Crossman that the then system of allocations was unfair, or perhaps to the academics who have made awkward comparisons.' (Anonymous, 1975b)

The first hospital revenue allocation formula was devised under Crossman's aegis progressively to equalise Regional hospital revenue budgets. The formula could not apply below RHB level because the HMCs responsible for running the hospitals below Regional level were not constituted with geographical, population responsibilities. The Crossman Formula was implemented by the Conservative administration under Crossman's successor, Sir Keith Joseph. In opposition, from 1970 to 1974, the Labour Party continued to discuss inequalities in the availability of Health Service resources and to put forward proposals for change which a future Labour Government might implement. By February 1974 when a Labour Government was returned to office, Regional inequalities were little changed. The new Minister of State for Health was David Owen, who rapidly became strongly influenced by the intellectual justification of the 1974 reorganisation to secure a more rational allocation of resources at all levels within the NHS, both between care groups and geographical areas. Owen also had access to his party's previous proposals on resource allocation developed during the period in opposition and to the views of the Secretary of State's Special Adviser, Professor Brian Abel-Smith. Abel-Smith, a social policy analyst in the Fabian tradition, had been a long-time proponent of a more rational formula for resource allocation, ever since his involvement in the research for the Guillebaud Committee in the mid-1950s. Owen was thus receptive to his DHSS Regional Group officials' own proposals for a major technical improvement in the methods of geographical resource allocation and obtained Cabinet support for the introduction of a system based on good socialist principles of equity and allocation in relation to need. Accordingly, the Secretary of State, Barbara Castle, agreed to establish the Resource Allocation Working Party. She was preoccupied with a host of other NHS problems including negotiations on a new consultants' contract and the furore generated by the decision to phase out pay beds from NHS hospitals and played little part in RAWP or its implementation.

Part of the explanation for David Owen's interest in geographical resource redistribution would also seem to lie in the political pushes and economic constraints faced by the new Labour Government. These have been analysed by Klein (1979). All Labour Ministers were under pressure from their supporters to satisfy left-wing aspirations for radical reform and from the trade unions to give social spending high priority in return for wage restraint; yet the Government had inherited a worsening economic situation where inflation and unemployment were rising rapidly. Easy assumptions of continued growth in the economy and public spending were coming to an end. DHSS Ministers' ability to improve the NHS in terms of increasing resources was thus severely limited by the poor state of the economy and further hampered by their decision to give first place to raising the wages and salaries of NHS employees ahead of improving service provision. Ministers faced a major presentational difficulty of how to formulate radical initiatives with little chance of obtaining extra resources. Klein argues that Barbara Castle's decision to pursue the issue of pay beds was directly related to the fact that abolishing pay beds appeared to have no visible economic cost consequences but was ideologically attractive to the Government's supporters, particularly the trade unions (Klein, 1979). In the same way, the emphasis given by David Owen to the need to redistribute resources within the NHS has been interpreted as a response to the fact that redistribution and "fair shares" did not seem so reliant on economic growth as a commitment to improve and enlarge the NHS and were thus attractive, egalitarian policies for a period of stringency (Pollitt, 1984, p. 52). Furthermore, Ministers were made aware by officials that some better form of control over the geographically unequal pattern of resource allocation would be required if their long-cherished policies to favour the "cinderella" care groups were to stand any chance of implementation on a near standstill NHS buget. However, when RAWP was set up in 1975 there was scant appreciation in DHSS of the future importance of rationing devices. A year later the situation had altered completely.

CONCLUSIONS

The detailed history of the origins of the RAWP has yet to be assembled. While the protagonists are still available for interview, the opportunity should be taken to document this major initiative more fully. The existing literature points to the main influences on policy and thinking before the setting up of the Working Party, but in no sense offers a full account. According to Christopher Pollitt, in the years 1974-5 leading directly to RAWP:

> 'Briefly, ... the circumstances had seemed similar to 1948: an energetic Labour Minister with equality high on his/her list of priorities; an economic crisis putting pressure on resources; a new organisational structure (the foundation of the NHS in 1948; its first major reorganisation in 1974).'
> (Pollitt, 1984, p. 52)

In Pollitt's view, such factors explain in broad terms why RAWP was convened in 1975. On the other hand, the profound differences between 1974-75 and 1948 explain why the formula itself was less radical and its implementation more limited than the changes brought about in 1948. For a start the Labour Government had a very small House of Commons majority, its manifesto was predominantly focused on economic and industrial policy and there was no spirit of post-war reconstruction for reformers to draw on (Pollitt, 1984, p. 52). In this context it is not surprising that the RAWP formula was explicitly aimed at geographical equality in resource availability rather than tackling the more controversial social class inequalities in health and health care utilisation, and that movement towards equality subsequently has been relatively slow.

Pollitt focuses predominantly on political and economic factors external to the Health Service and the DHSS in explaining the convening of RAWP. Yet there is little evidence that any of the factors he mentions, aside from the 1974 reorganisation were important in the decision to set up RAWP. By contrast, and more convincingly, Ham (1985, pp. 123-4) interprets the establishment of RAWP as the result of an internal DHSS initiative in which civil servants were the primary source of political change acting on a receptive Minister, David Owen. In addition, the work of a number of outside advisers and researchers is credited with influence both on civil servants and Ministers. Ham quotes the Crossman Diaries which show senior civil servants presenting papers to the Secretary of State on Regional inequalities in the availability of health service resources as far back as July 1969. The redistributive implications were made plain to Crossman and emerge in paragraph 79 of Crossman's 1970 Green Paper on the future organisation of the Health Service which sets out a system of allocations based on the needs of administrative populations (DHSS, 1970a). RAWP can thus be seen as the culmination of a series of discussions between civil servants, health policy experts and Ministers stretching back to the Guillebaud Committee in the mid-1950s. This long internal genesis may also explain, in part, RAWP's longevity as a policy since 1976, although other factors have been important. Firstly, by concentrating on geographical inequalities of resource inputs and by setting a relatively modest pace of change, the orginators of the RAWP process were able to secure for it the support of successive Secretaries of State both Labour and Conservative from 1976 to date. Secondly, by involving senior NHS managers in its construction, the DHSS was able to reduce opposition to the new methods in the NHS. Thirdly, RAWP was explicitly formulated to create equal opportunity of access to services for those in equal need. This was in the tradition of the original NHS Act of 1946 and did not include any mechanism actively to secure equality of access. The resulting consensus surrounding the broad objectives of RAWP is notable. However, every other aspect of RAWP, both conceptually and technically, beyond the simple belief in "fair shares", has been the subject of continuous criticism and debate since 1976. The rest of this review covers these controversies.

PART ONE

THE POPULATION AND POPULATION WEIGHTINGS

CHAPTER THREE

DEFINING THE POPULATION BASE

POPULATION DATA

Significance of Population Data

The population base used in the calculation of RAWP targets has been relatively little discussed in the literature, yet the population base is the main determinant of the size of the RAWP target at Regional level and in most Districts. This highlights the need for accurate and reliable population statistics. By comparison inaccuracies in morbidity, utilisation and cost data have far less impact on targets. Errors in the calculation of the population base have a fundamental and unambiguous impact on targets (Holland, Charlton, Patrick and West, 1980). Furthermore it is a matter of concern to select the most appropriate measure of population from those available given expected trends and patterns of migration. The ideal would be to have access to data from an annual as opposed to the customary decennial national Census of population. Between Censuses, annual present population estimates are made which lack the reliability of a recent Census, For example, Holland et al (1980, p.iv) report a possible 5% cumulative error between the Office of Population Censuses and Surveys' (OPCS) population estimate for 1970 for an AHA and the population from the 1971 Census, due to nine years' worth of unreported migration. This would amount to a fundamental error in any potential RAWP target calculation, bound to overshadow all other possible revisions in components of the formula. Although District targets are not so uniformly dominated by the population component in the RAWP formula as Regional targets are, this example shows how changes in the smaller populations at District level, or especially those characteristics which most affect weightings, can lead to wide fluctuations in targets (Paton, 1985, p.12). Population information at District level, whether projections or current estimates is more precarious than at RHA level, particularly in Districts which are not coterminous with their local authorities. Reasonably reliable estimates of local authority populations are available. On the other hand, the use of population projections in resource allocation also has its hazards, since projections rely on assumptions about trends in fertility, mortality and migration extrapolated from past behaviour.

RAWP Recommendations for the Population Base of Targets

For revenue targets RAWP recommended that the calculation of the targets should be based upon 'the estimate of the mid-year population of each Region nearest to the year for which allocations are made'. The same base was to be used by Regions in the calculation of AHA revenue targets. In practice each annual allocation would be based on the mid-year estimate of the population level two years earlier (DHSS 1976c, pp.13-14, para. 2.2). For capital, RAWP recommended that a five-year forward projection of population be used as the basis for calculations in national RAWP, in order to match population to the likely time when capital projects would first come into use (DHSS, 1976c, p.64, para. 5.6.1).

Criticisms of the RAWP Methods

The main criticism of the RAWP method of establishing a base population for revenue targets concerned the inevitable time lag of two to two and a half years between the year of the population estimate and the year for which allocations were being made. The main complaints came from Regions such as East Anglia and Oxford with fast-growing populations. Winyard (1981) showed that the RAWP approach penalised Regions with rapidly growing populations and argued that some form of population projections shoud be used. RAWP's approach was unfair because it meant that Regions losing population were continuing to be provided with funds for populations they no longer had, while the Regions gaining population had insufficient resources to meet population needs. Worse than this, Regions losing population could even continue to receive increasing allocations as a result of an inflated target population. Some critics argued that New Towns and areas of known future population expansion should be provided with health facilities in advance of the arrival of the population. Similar critiscisms were voiced sub-Regionally. On capital RAWP, the main criticism was to point out the seven-year discrepancy between the population bases of revenue and capital targets. Buxton and Klein argued that this could cause problems in phasing the revenue and capital requirements of new developments (Royal Commission on the National Health Service, 1978b, p.10).

In response to these criticisms the Joint Working Group (JWG) of the Thames Regions and DHSS on resource allocation in the four Thames RHAs recommended that at AHA level in the Thames Regions the population base should be the latest estimate of the mid-year population nearest to the year for which targets rather than allocations were calculated (DHSS and Thames Regional Health Authorities, 1979). The JWG was sceptical of the use of population projections, as was the Advisory Group on Resource Allocation (AGRA) appointed at the same period to review key aspects of the national RAWP formula. The AGRA was against projections because they were based on assumptions, they were not produced annually and they were liable to serious error. It was felt at the time that population estimates were the most reliable figures available and had the advantage of being produced each year based on records of actual numbers of births and deaths. Additionally, regardless of the accuracy of projections, AGRA was worried that their use in RAWP would obscure the need to take account of the necessary time-lag between a Region or Area losing population and its consequent ability to release NHS resources. Projections would place even greater strain on the RAWP "losers". AGRA believed that the special needs of Regions with fast-growing populations shoud be taken into account by DHSS on an ad hoc basis when deciding the precise level of actual annual allocations. Unlike the JWG, AGRA recommended no change at all in the population base for revenue targets, not even the use of an estimate nearest to the year for which targets were calculated. Capital targets were already based on a projection of population for 5 years' ahead and thus AGRA saw no need to change this either (DHSS, 1980b).

Population Projections for the Year of Allocation

Since the AGRA report, criticisms of the use of population estimates have continued from those Regions with expanding populations. As a result of this pressure DHSS has modified its approach from 1985/86 in consultation with Regional Treasurers. Population projections for the mid-point of the year of allocation are now used as the base population data in national RAWP for calculating Regional targets (DHSS, 1984a). Under the former system 1985/86 targets would have been calculated using OPCS mid-1983 population estimates.

Under the new system, population projections for mid-1985 based on the 1981 Census population were used. This reform has gone some way to meeting the complaints of Wessex, East Anglia and Oxford (Winyard, 1981).

Coping with Long-Term Shifts in Populations

The use of population projections for the year of allocation as the base for calculating revenue targets is a sensible way of responding to rapid shifts of population over a relatively short time-span. However, it still leaves unresolved a further problem of how to take account of long-term population movements in changing the pattern of NHS resource distribution. This was first raised in Winyard's original criticism of RAWP's revenue target population base (Winyard, 1981). As the under-target Regions progressively move nearer to target, future changes in their populations become ever more important to anticipate so as to avoid a situation in which resources are reallocated to Regions where the population has very recently declined. For example, at the end of 1985/6, Northern Region was 3% below target and North Western Region 1.8% below target (DHSS, 1985b). OPCS forecasts that the total population of the two Regions will decline by 2.6% and 2% respectively by 1991 and by 4.1% and 2.7% by 2001 (Office of Population Censuses and Surveys, 1983). There is a risk that as the long-term drift of population to the South East continues population will be moving in the opposite direction to RAWP redistribution. It would be unfortunate to have to reverse the RAWP process for a Region which had very recently reached its target and it may be difficult to do so, because much of the differential growth in the Northern, North Western and Trent Regions has tended to be invested in hospitals which are relatively inflexible in reallocation terms. Thus there may be a problem in the future, of hospitals in the north of England without the resident population to justify their existence, while in the South and East, especially in the "microchip belt" around the Thames valley, there is a lack of accessible hospital beds. The degree of redistributive flexibility will depend on whether growth allocations are primarily invested in conventional hospital provision or in alternative modes of care. As hospitals become increasingly productive with lower lengths of stay and an increasing proportion of day care and outpatient work, it may well be that fewer hospitals and fewer beds are required. It may be possible to encourage RAWP-gaining Regions and Districts to invest in staff, particularly in the priority care groups in a way which does not build historical rigidity into the health care system. On the other hand, traditionally "deprived" Regions and Districts are likely to interpret their own intests differently and choose to invest in provision which cannot so easily be wrested away from them.

In the light of the above discussion and given that targets are supposed to be guides to medium to long-term, future changes in resources, it would seem more logical to base them on projections of future populations for the years to which the targets refer and to relate actual allocations to these targets rather than to base targets on calculations of current population for the year of allocation. This change could mean a reduction in the scale of redistribution to Regions and Districts currently deemed under-target. Under such a system the choice of target year could be critical and would become a source of political debate within the NHS. The further into the future, the more it would benefit the South and East, but on the basis of less reliable population projections.

ESTIMATING CROSS-BOUNDARY FLOWS

RAWP Recommendations for Estimating Cross-Boundary Flows

The general principle guiding RAWP was one of capitation-based finance. RAWP assumed that equity was best defined in terms of the geographical redistribution of resources so that provision should be physically equalised in relation to the needs of resident populations in each part of the country. Given the knowledge available about the effect of distance on access and utilisation, an administrative definition of equity based on boundaries was sensible. Each Region or Area was to receive funding in relation to the size and needs of the population defined by its administrative boundaries and was then requried to manage services for that population within the sum made available. In theory, this principle implies a system which would ignore the existence of patients who live in one administrative unit but are treated in another and which would aim swiftly to eliminate such flows. Indeed, the use of residential populations does appear to be a sensible basis for determining the 10% or so of expenditure on community health services in the RAWP formula. However for provision such as acute hospital services and mental illness and mental handicap services, RAWP identified major practical obstacles to this simple approach. RAWP recognised that in many situations, particularly sub-Regionally, the historic imbalance of service availability was too great for extensive cross-boundary flows to be eliminated except in the very long term and that it was not necessarily desirable, feasible, or affordable for all AHAs and Districts to pursue policies of complete self-sufficiency. Historically, hospitals had never been limited to specific catchments and GPs were sure to resist interference with their freedom to refer their patients to the hospital and consultant of their choosing. Furthermore, the fact that AHAs were intended from 1974 to provide a comprehensive range of services did not and could not have meant an all-embracing range of services. Thus flows were envisaged continuing (even after considerable redistribution) because of unavoidable gaps in local provision, factors of patient convenience and clinical freedom of referral. The Working Party assumed that RHAs would make judgements about flows of convenience and those caused by inadequate services and plan developments accordingly. As a result, RAWP opted to take existing patient flows into account when calculating revenue targets so that Regions and Areas would be funded on the basis of populations served. (No allowances for cross-boundary flows were made in capital RAWP). RAWP judged it senseless, as well as too costly and difficult, to equalise on the basis of AHA or District self-sufficiency. Thus an activity element, in the form of an allowance for existing flows of inpatients, was introduced into the RAWP target calculation, which was theoretically based on the different principle of finance by capitation.

Although RAWP's decision to compromise on its geographical, administrative definition of equity may have been sensible in itself, it demanded a further logical step; namely to examine which of the existing cross-boundary flows were publicly acceptable, which were the result of scarcity, which the result of convenience and which imposed excessive costs on consumers in terms of travel time or inconvenience and to take decisions to alter or maintain flows, accordingly. The significance of the need to make judgements about flows was perhaps not fully appreciated at the time by RAWP which effectively treated flows as immutable "facts of life". The Working Party's primary focus was on the process of redistribution between Regions. At this level, patient flows were relatively small and tended to be self-cancelling in their overall impact on Regional targets and allocations. Thus the allowance for cross-boundary flows was no more than a minor adjustment to the formula. Subsequently, critics have tended to agree with this judgement. At Regional level, targets are robust to changes in flow calculations (Senn and Shaw, 1978). However, sub-Regionally, patients flow extensively across administrative divisions, especially in the cities and crossboundary flow adjustments can form a major element in the composition of targets. At this level, the RAWP method of calculating catchment populations for different components in the formula has been the focus for extensive debate. The majority of the criticism has been technical and focused on the cross-boundary flow adjustment itself. However, underlying RAWP's decision to accommodate the existing pattern of flows within a policy of redistribution lie far more wide-ranging issues concerning the best way of implementing objectives of an equitable and efficient health system. For example, recent discussion centres on whether quasi-market mechanisms such as cross-charging are more likely to bring about an equitable provision of efficiently run health services than more conventional approaches based on strategic planning. This sort of debate concerns fundamental issues about how best to generate appropriate managerial and clinical incentives in a socialised health system. It is explored in Chapter Six.

To compensate and debit Regions (and by implication, sub-Regionally also) for cross-boundary flows of non-psychiatric inpatients, RAWP chose to reduce or increase the non-psychiatric impatient (NPIP) weighted population depending on whether the Region (or AHA) was a net importer or exporter of patients using the method of calculating catchment populations known as Net Flow. The patient flows used for the calculation of catchments were derived from Hospital Activity Analysis (HAA). Net Flow is perhaps the simplest method of calculating catchments. It adds to the resident population of a Region or District the net inflow of patients multiplied by a factor representing the population equivalent (or value) of each case (ie. the total population divided by the total number of cases). Another way of presenting the method is:

$$\text{Residential Population} + \frac{\text{Net inflow of patients}}{\text{National admission rate}}$$

In detail, the national RAWP method uses HAA data for each Region on the numbers of episodes of inpatient treatment by specialty generated by people from each of the other 13 Regions, to calculate patient flows in broad groups of specialties. The net cost of flows is determined by applying the national average cost per case for each group to the appropriate net flow figures. The resultant adjustments in expenditure are converted into population equivalents by reference to the national average cost per head of population on NPIP services and applied to the appropriate weighted population for each Region (DHSS, 1976c, Annex C, pp. 103-107, paras. C11-C13.2). The calculation thus depends on the relationship of local admission rates to the national admission rate. However, RAWP recommended that flows should be allowed for in targets at national average specialty costs rather than local costs (DHSS, 1976c, p.22, para. 2.17). The RAWP credit for cross-boundary flows is not immediate and it is not direct, for three reasons. Firstly, in any year, compensation is made for flows which took place two years earlier. Secondly, it is made in the form of a notional population rather than cash (although sub-Regionally it is usually now in cash) and thirdly, it represents an adjustment to the ten-year target rather than to the current allocation.

Although there has been considerable criticism of the adequacy of using national average costs by specialty in cross-boundary flow adjustments (the debate is covered in Chapter Six, 'Managing Cross-boundary Flows of Patients And the Pursuit of Equity'), the method of calculating the population equivalent of flows has far greater impact on the eventual size of RAWP targets than modifications to the costing of flows. However, RAWP recognised the possible limitations of national average specialty costs and drew attention to the importance of developing improved systems for costing patient care both for services to residents and cross-boundary flows (DHSS, 1976c, p.82, para. 6.24).

RAWP was unable to include an allowance for cross-boundary flows of outpatients and day cases except in the case of formal agency arrangements, because there were no generally available statistics. This represents a sizeable omission since the outpatient and day case component is second only to the NPIP component in its contribution to the final target in most health authorities. The Working Party was unable to identify a suitable proxy indicator. It was not possible to assume with any confidence that the known pattern of inpatient flows would correspond with the pattern of outpatient and day case flows. RAWP concluded that there was an urgent need to assemble better information on day and outpatient service flows, which were particularly important in sub-Regional calculations. Day and outpatient services represented a substantial and growing proportion of NHS expenditure (DHSS, 1976c, p.23, para. 2.18.3). The SHARE formula in Scotland included an outpatient and day services cross-boundary flow allowance, but only by assuming the same pattern of flows as for inpatients (Scottish Home and Health Department, 1977).

For the community health services component, RAWP was again unable to include a cross-boundary flow adjustment for lack of the necessary data. However this omission was not serious since these services comprise a far smaller proportion of total expenditure and are generally provided on the basis of residential population with few if any cross-boundary flows.

In the mental illness and mental handicap hospital inpatient services components of the revenue target, adjustments for cross-boundary flows were an important element in District targets and allocations because of the historical tendency for many Districts to rely on hospital inpatient facilities provided in other Areas or Districts. The compensation for flows in the original report comprised two parts. For short-stay, acute patients the Net Flow method was used in the same way as in the NPIP component and subject to the same criticisms (see below). For long-stay patients RAWP did not have data on patients' origins and thus flow adjustments to the weighted residential population were calculated on the basis of the observed number of cases treated in the District versus the number which would have been expected from national average hospitalisation rates given the size and age/sex structure of the resident population. The difference in caseload was converted to a population equivalent by multiplying by the relevant national average costs for either long-stay mental illness or mental handicap patients, summarising the resulting costs and dividing by the national average cost per head of population on long-stay mental illness or mental handicap patients (DHSS, 1976c, Annex C, pp.115-C117, paras. C21-C22.4). In effect the original RAWP method set targets for mental illness and mental handicap services based on inpatient activity rates. As a result there was a disincentive to the development of desired community care alternatives to hospitalisation, since a patient discharged into "community care" would represent a deduction from a Region's target at the rate of the average inpatient cost per case. The planning implications of RAWP methods in mental illness and mental handicap are covered more fully in Chapter Seven 'RAWP and Planning'. In order to overcome this disincentive to good practice many Regions which now have access to data on patient origin, have developed sub-Regional funding methods which explicitly charge user Districts as long as their residents remain in other Districts' hospitals.

Criticisms of RAWP Recommendations for Estimating the Extent of Cross-Boundary Flows - Alternative Methods of Calculating Catchment Populations

As soon as RAWP reported it was criticised for its use of the Net Flow method of calculating the flow adjustment to the NPIP residential population. Criticisms focused particularly on the sub-Regional level where flow adjustments formed a far more significant part of targets than at Regional level. Regional targets are likely to be robust with respect to the choice of method of estimating flow adjustments to populations, since the proportion of the final target contributed by the flow adjustment is dwarfed by the contribution of the residential component of the target. Adjustment using the Net Flow method appears to achieve reasonable results at this level.

In using a Net Flow adjustment RAWP was in fact estimating AHA and District catchment populations. Yet the method of Proportionate Flow not Net Flow was regarded by many commentators at the time as the standard (and therefore, by implication, best) method since it was generally used in analysing HAA for the calculation of catchment populations for planning purposes. At first sight, estimating cross-boundary flows and thereby calculating catchment populations seems a straightforward solution to the problem of adjusting residential populations for flows; the only obstacle being the selection of technically the best method of estimation. The purpose of using catchment populations in RAWP targets was to have a method which could be used in the presence of large cross-boundary flows to provide a way of correcting inequalities in the current consumption of services. RAWP chose Net Flow. However, there is no consensus on how catchment populations should be calculated. Since 1976, Regions have used a variety of alternative methods to calculate catchment populations in response to perceived weaknesses of Net Flow sub-Regionally for calculating AHA and DHA targets. The range of available methods with the exception of Ebb and Flow, is well set out in Beech, Craig and Bevan (1987). Unfortunately the estimation of catchment populations, regardless of the method chosen, is most controversial when most needed, ie., in the presence of large flows and inequalities in consumption (Beech, Craig and Bevan, 1987). In these circumstances different methods give different results. The calculation of catchment populations is only straightforward where there is equality of use of services by residents of Districts, in which case there is no point in bothering with cross-boundary flow calculations (Senn and Shaw, 1978)! In reality, of course, in most Regions there is considerable inequality in the use of services in relation to need and often extensive flows.

A number of different methods other than RAWP's choice, Net Flow, are currently in use by Regions to describe catchment populations for resource allocation. This can lead to inconsistencies between Regions with the possibility that flows between two adjacent Districts in different Regions will be treated in three ways: by the Net Flow method used in national RAWP; and by the two methods to estimate catchment populations by the two Regions (Brazier, 1986).

Commonly, the solution to the problem of adjusting populations for flows is seen in terms of identifying the most accurate method of calculating catchment populations. Pinder (1982) described six methods of calculating catchment populations for sub-Regional resource allocation and explored their relative accuracy:

1. Resident Population (used for community health services where there were no data on attendance patterns);

2. Workload method, which distributes the total Regional population in proportion to the workload in each District (extensively used for funding outpatient services when patient data on place of residence are not available);

3. Proportionate Flow method, a disaggregation of the workload method which distributes the resident population of each District in proportion to their place of treatment;

4. Net Flow method, which adds to the resident population the net inflow multiplied by a factor representing the population equivalent or value of each case (used in National RAWP);

5. Ebb and Flow method, which consists of the resident population of a District, multiplied by the number of cases treated in the District, divided by the total number of cases from the District (used in at least one Region (Cottrell, 1979a));

6.   Treatment Intensity method, which distributes the catchment population of
     each District in proportion to where they live.

Using data from a hypothetical Region, Pinder (1982) demonstrated that each
method produces   the   same   results   only when the admission rates of the
constituent DHAs are   equal.   When admission rates vary, the results of the
different methods vary.   Pinder attempted to see which method gave the most
"accurate" estimation of catchment populations by assuming that the most
accurate result was the one produced when District admission rates were equal;
ie. which method is most stable in the face of random fluctuations in caseloads
and   flows?   He ran sufficient simulations with random alterations in caseload
data to build up measures of their relative effect on catchments using different
methods of calculation. In an important finding, he showed that the "accuracy"
of all the methods (except residential population) was found to deteriorate as a
function of increasing admission rate variation and increasing proportionate
cross-boundary flows. However, the Net Flow method selected by RAWP appeared to
give the "best" (most stable) estimates in the simulation exercise.

While Pinder (1982) appeared to favour Net Flow as the most stable of the
available methods of calculation of catchments, Senn and Shaw (1978) favoured
Proportionate Flow (which allocates local population to the health authorities
serving a locality in proportion to the total cases treated by those health
authorities) over Net Flow on the grounds that with Proportionate Flow, however
high or low the admission rate in any given locality, the total population
allocated from that locality to the health authority of residence and to other
health authorities always had to equal the population of the locality.   This
contrasts with Net Flow where the higher the <u>local</u> admission rate, the greater
the population credited and vice-versa. Thus an admission rate above the
national average is likely to produce an over-estimate of flows. Since
differences in admission rates between Districts are likely to reflect different
levels of past provision, Senn and Shaw (1978) criticised Net Flow as likely to
perpetuate or even exacerbate inequalities in provision since it effectively
freezes the pattern of flows. They concluded that at sub-Regional level flows
are too important to be dealt with crudely by adjusting resident populations by
Net Flow as RAWP recommended.   They outline an approach which would calculate
catchment populations <u>prospectively</u> basing them on future plans for capital
developments aimed at equalising the availability and consumption of services,
rather than on data on past (unequal) usage of services as in RAWP.

In fact Senn and Shaw's (1978) criticism of Net Flow for penalising Districts
with poor facilities and rewarding those with good facilities also applies to
Proportionate Flow according to Gandy (1979b). Districts with poor facilities
tend to have lower admission rates than better provided Districts. The effect
of this under Proportionate Flow is to reduce the denominator in the calculation
which means that the lower the admission rate in one District, the higher the
population credit to another District for each patient treated outside the
District. The converse is likely to happen in a well-provided District.
However, in the context of RAWP redistribution, this pattern of incentives may
be desirable to stimulate an equitable use of resources.

The above problems with the calculation of catchment populations in the presence
of inequalities in utilisation rates, are not confined to the methods of Net
Flow and Proportionate Flow. All the methods are controversial when flows are
large and inequalities in consumption are pronounced. Beech, Craig and Bevan
(1987) demonstrate that for a hypothetical RHA of two Districts, with unequal
resource consumption by residents, the Net Flow, Proportionate Flow and
Treatment Intensity methods each produces different population results, which in
turn, have a major impact on consequent RAWP targets. Applying the three
methods to Districts in South East Thames RHA and calculating RAWP targets

accordingly, the authors produce a variation in District targets by up to 16% between the three methods. The reason for the difference in results between methods lies in the fact that each makes different assumptions about how past statistics of flows can be used to determine the sizes of the adjustments to residential populations, which are then used to derive targets for future allocations.

Although individual Regions have disagreed since 1976 on which method of calculating catchment populations is best, they have concurred in assuming that the solution to the problem of dealing with patient flows across administrative boundaries in a system of geographical resource allocation lies in calculating catchment populations which are descriptive estimates of past patterns of flows. Beech, Craig and Bevan (1987) question this. They consider whether any of the methods can lead to sub-Regional equity (for example, in terms of equalising hospitalisation rates) and if so, under what assumptions, and in turn, whether these assumptions are sensible. They conclude that the assumptions required by each of the methods are dubious and therefore that none of the methods is satisfactory to enable Districts to plan an equitable distribution of services by estimating the needs of catchment populations.

They contend that a satisfactory method of estimating catchments for RAWP has to produce targets which enable Districts to achieve equity. This will only be achieved if the predictions about flows implicit in each method are fulfilled. Accordingly, they test each of the available methods for inclusion in RAWP on the basis of three criteria: whether or not it embodies sensible assumptions as to how Districts should move towards equity; whether or not it is likely to model clinicians' and patients' future behaviour correctly. The nub of their critique is that catchment populations, however calculated, are essentially descriptive means of accounting for past flows. They are inadequate for predicting the pattern of flows which will result from a process of future resource redistribution. Using a hypothetical two District Region, Beech et al (1987) modelled the effect of changes in allocations on inter-District flows and found that Net Flow was likely to lead to a 'spiral of decline' in inner city Districts which have large cross-boundary flows, since the Net Flow method assumes that cross-boundary flows will remain constant. Thus, under Net Flow, as over-target DHAs reduce their expenditure, more of their residents are likely to seek treatment in adjacent DHAs. These extra outflows will cause targets to fall still further fuelling a 'spiral of decline'. Beech et al found that under the assumptions implicit in Proportionate Flow, over-target Districts were required to reduce the services to their residents while expanding them for non-residents in order to move towards equity and avoid a 'spiral of decline'. It would seem unrealistic for local management to contemplate such a discretionary admissions policy.

In certain respects the Treatment Intensity method appeared the most reasonable in that it allowed Districts to move towards target by modifying their capacity to treat, but while continuing to admit patients under the former unplanned access policies. There was no need to be selective. This method was recommended by the Acute Services Working Group of the Joint Group on Performance Indicators as the approved method of calculating catchment populations for DHSS Performance Indicators (DHSS, 1984b). However, the Treatment Intensity method assumes that the mix of patients treated in a District in terms of District of origin will remain the same throughout the redistributive process. Beech et al contend that this is unlikely. They also point out that the degree of change in the volume of flows indicated by Treatment Intensity to achieve equity (in terms of hospitalisation rates) is based solely on the solution of a mathematical equation. Thus the method is less stable than the Net Flow method and vulnerable to manipulation through the way in which flows are reported. However, all the other methods are also vulnerable to this latter criticism to varying degrees.

CONCLUSIONS

The conclusion to be drawn from this discussion of the merits of using alternative methods to Net Flow to calculate cross-boundary flow adjustments in RAWP is that far from simply being a technical matter, all current methods contain inherent assumptions about what will happen as Districts move to targets which are unlikely to make sense to those involved. For example, it seems politically unrealistic to expect Districts not to protect services to their residents. The proponents of the various methods start from the assumption that it is possible to extrapolate from past flow data what the future use of servies will be and thereby secure equity. However, Beech, Craig and Bevan (1987) succeed in showing that the methods fail to provide a credible model of future cross-boundary flows because they cannot take adequate account of what a series of inter-related DHAs, their clinicians and their GPs, would do in conditions of uncertainty and financial redistribution. In particular, none of the available methods of calculating catchment populations for RAWP can overcome the fact that Districts with large cross-boundary flows which are expected to reduce their residents' use of services in order to meet their RAWP targets, are handicapped by having very limited control over their residents' use of services in other Districts. This can lead to the absurd situation in which the most effective way for an over-target District to reach its target would be to refuse to treat any of its residents at its hospitals and to treat only in-flows from other Districts.

Thus it can be seen that the apparently straightforward matter of adjusting the population base for flows when setting RAWP targets based oncOCe principle of finance by capitation, raises far wider questions about whether the implicit incentives generated for DHAs by sub-Regional RAWP are managerially sensible. Are there better ways of securing the transition from an inequitable to an equitable pattern of resource distribution and utilisation in relation to need where flows are such an important feature of Health Service activity? This theme is picked up again in Chapters Six and Seven which consider alternative ways of coping with flows while moving towards equity.

CHAPTER FOUR

MORTALITY, MORBIDITY AND THE NEED FOR HEALTH CARE

INTRODUCTION: THE METHOD OF WEIGHTING THE POPULATION FOR NEED

One of the main problems faced by RAWP in its capitation-based approach to the
allocation of resources was how to assess the health care needs of different
populations to establish the appropriate share of resources which each Region
and Area should receive. The Working Party recommended that the same principles
should be used for allocations at Regional and sub-Regional levels.   The
starting point was an estimate of the resources which would be allocated if the
population concerned used resources at the national average rate for the
relevant Service Category. However the relative health status and composition
of a population, as well as its sheer size affects its comparative need for
health care. Thus the population for each of the seven Service Categories used
in the RAWP revenue formula (1. Non-psychiatric inpatient services; 2.   out
and day patient services; 3.   community services; 4. ambulance services; 5.
family practitioner committee administration (excluded from 1982); 6.   mental
illness hospital inpatient services, and 7. mental handicap hospital inpatient
services) was adjusted to reflect likely differences in need in five ways by
taking into account:

1. age and sex structure of the population in the form of the national
    utilisation rates for each age and sex group (except for ambulance services
    and FPC administration);

2. mortality in the form of SMRs (standardised mortality ratios) except for
    mental illness, mental handicap and FPC administration;

3. fertility rates for conditions associated with pregnancy;

4. martial status for mental illness inpatients;

5. cross boundary-flows of patients.

The resulting weighted populations for each Service Category were then to be
combined in proportion to the historic revenue expenditure on each Service
Category to produce a weighted population.   If appropriate, the population was
further adjusted for London weighting on salaries. An overall revenue 'target'
for redistributive change was then produced by dividing the resources available
nationally in proportion to each Region's weighted population. In turn, each
Region calculated AHA targets in proportion to each AHA population according to
its own modified version of the RAWP formula.

The status of the population weightings has been central to much of the
technical debate about RAWP, none more so than the decision to use SMRs to take
account of factors other than the age and sex composition of the population in
the calculation of both revenue and capital targets. In the Interim Report of

the Resource Allocation Working Party (August 1975) (DHSS, 1976c, Annex B, pp.93-6) Regional inpatient and outpatient caseloads were used as an indicator of need in addition to the national utilisation of services by age and sex groups. By the time of the final report, the caseload weighting had been rejected as inadequate since it tended to reflect need in terms of the available supply of services and an allowance for morbidity over and above the age/sex structure of the population had been included in the form of SMRs. RAWP proposed that for allocations to Regions SMRs should be used as follows in the calculation of the revenue target:

1. For ambulance services the crude population should be multiplied by the overall Regional SMR;

2. For day outpatient and community services the age/sex utilisation weighted population should be multiplied by the overall Regional SMR;

3. For non-psychiatric inpatient services (the largest single Service Category in terms of expenditure) the condition-specific age/sex utilisation weighted population should be multiplied by condition-specific age/sex Regional SMRs (the conditions were grouped under the 17 Chapters of the International Classification of Diseases.

Since mortality is the main weighting factor which varies appreciably between Regions after the age/sex composition of the population, the inclusion of SMRs had a greater impact on the relative position of Regions than any of the other changes made between the 1975 and 1976 reports, exceeding the effect of omitting the caseload factor and the inclusion of the Service Increment for Teaching (SIFT). Barr and Logan (1977) agreed with RAWP (DHSS, 1976c, p.84, para. 6.31) that this was the most important addition to the RAWP methodology contained in the final report. Introduction of a morbidity factor based on SMRs affected North Western, East Anglia, Mersey and Oxford particularly. Under the system based on the Interim Report, Oxford RHA was deemed to be just 'below target' but after allowance for SMRs it moved to being an 'over-target' Region. Mersey RHA moved in the opposite direction from substantially 'over-target' to 'under target' after the application of SMRs. This occurred because the final formula combined average bed utilisation and SMRs by ICD Chapter and thus the results were influenced by those groups of conditions having a high bed usage. Mersey had above average SMRs for most conditions, the highest being for conditions responsible for about one-third of national bed utilisation in general hospitals. By contrast Oxford had below average SMRs for most conditions, particularly those which had a high bed usage (DHSS, 1976c, p.77, para. 6.7).

Before discussing the extensive literature commenting on the use of SMRs in RAWP, it may be helpful to describe the thinking which lay behind the decision and RAWP's own analysis of the problem of quantifying the impact of morbidity on the need for health care. (The discussion which follows in the remainder of this Chapter refers to the use of SMRs in measuring health need in the non-psychiatric inpatient component of the RAWP revenue target, unless stated to the contrary).

RAWP'S JUSTIFICATION FOR THE USE OF SMRS

RAWP's aim was to ensure that resources are made available to enable health authorities to meet the needs arising from the morbidity of the populations they serve. Thus morbidity variations had to be incorporated in the resource allocation procedure. The Working Party recognised that in many conditions, morbidity and mortality rates are probably not significantly influenced by the intervention of health services and that redistribution of resources may not therefore have a significant impact on morbidity. 'But this cannot be a reason for ignoring them [morbidity characteristics], since the NHS has a statutory responsibility to respond to the needs which those characteristics generate' (DHSS, 1976c, p.84, para. 6.31). Furthermore, RAWP argued that there were certain activities for which health authorities had a responsibility such as preventive measures and promoting environmental improvements, which could influence morbidity, and which it asserted were needed more in areas with greater morbidity and mortality. The Working Party held that since the majority of the commonest conditions leading to use of health services showed little geographical variation in incidence, the main determinants of need for health care lay in the age/sex structure of a population. Yet the Working Party was also aware that there were certain frequently occurring conditions which displayed a very marked geographical variation (eg. chronic bronchitis, cancer and coronary heart disease which account for over half of all deaths). It was thus justifiable to provide more resources in those areas where needs were likely to be greater as revealed in morbidity statistics after the age/sex structure of the population had been accounted for.

The problem facing RAWP was that no widely accepted, tailor-made morbidity measure existed for resource allocation purposes. In the Interim Report (1975) RAWP had used Regional inpateint and outpatient caseloads as an indicator of relative need for hospital inpatient services over and above that arising from the age/sex structure of the population. The Working Party was determined to replace this indicator with one far less influenced by the supply of hospital facilities and considered a range of possible morbidity indicators (DHSS, 1976c, pp. 14-22, paras. 2.5-2.15). Sickness absence statistics derived from DHSS sickness benefit records were rejected because they did not cover children, the elderly and many married women; they related to the structure of industry in different Regions; and were primarily a measure of need for GP not hospital care. Self-reported sickness data from the General Household Survey (GHS) were rejected because the GHS sample was not drawn to relate to NHS boundaries and yielded very small numbers sub-Regionally; self-reported sickness was not necessarily a measure of need for formal health care; differences in the levels of self-reported sickness might be partly due to differences in perception and reporting of sickness; (for example, the certified sickness absence rates for Wales are consistently higher than for the remainder of Great Britain - in 1973/74 the average days certified incapacity per man at risk in Wales was double that for England and Wales (Dowie, 1978, p.61)); diagnostic data would not be accurate enough for resource allocation; and collecting survey data on sickness at local level would be costly.

Mortality statistics were then considered as a possible proxy indicator of morbidity. The advantages of mortality data were perceived to be:

1. comprehensive coverage;

2. regular availability at all levels of NHS;

3. able to be compiled by place of residence;

4. high quality and reliability;

5. able to be related to diagnostic conditions by age and sex groups in a a way other sources could not;

6. independent of supply.

At Regional level, SMRs varied by 28% for males and 21% for females. Although RAWP did not have good evidence which explained this variation, the Working Party:

'... believed that Regional differences in morbidity explain the greater
part of it [differential Regional mortality] and that statistics of
relative differences in Regional morbidity, if they existed, would exhibit
the same pattern as those for mortality.'
(DHSS, 1976c, p.16, para. 2.8)

Without reporting the actual correlations, the RAWP report included four maps of
England and Wales which compared Regional SMRs divided into three bands ("high",
"medium" and "low") with similar maps of certified spells of sickness incapacity
and self-reported acute and chronic illness from the GHS by Region, also divided
into "high", "medium" and "low" categories. The reader was expected to infer
the correlations by eye and take on trust that, 'the comparison reveals
significant positive correlations' (DHSS, 1976c, p.16, para. 2.9) between
Regional differences in mortality and the chosen morbidity measures. On the
basis of this evidence, mortality was judged the best available indicator of
geographical variations in morbidity except for pregnancy and diseases of the
skin. The use of mortality and morbidity indicators together was rejected
because it was believed that this would result in 'double counting'. Yet as we
shall see the data concerning the adequacy of mortality as a proxy for morbidity
can be interpreted differently. The relationship between mortality and
different types of morbidity and therefore of the need for health services is
more complex than RAWP admitted (Walker, 1978).

In order to use the mortality statistics to relate Regional variations in
morbidity to the actual need for health care for non-psychiatric inpatient
services RAWP chose to group the causes of death according to the seventeen
Chapters of the ICD (omitting conditions with very few deaths) and calculated
the demand for health care generated by each Chapter using the national age-sex
hospital bed usage rates for each Chapter. The resultant weightings were then
combined with the weightings derived from the SMRs for the same ICD Chapters to
produce a set of weighting factors independent of Regional differences in the
supply of NHS facilities and in the view of RAWP, reflecting morbidity
differences between different parts of the country, over and above those
resulting from the age and sex structure of populations. 'The method ensures
that, in applying SMRs by condition, account is taken of the proportionate
national bed utilisation for each condition' (DHSS, 1976c, p.21, para. 2.12).

For derivation of AHA/District revenue targets RAWP recommended in principle,
applying the same methods used at national level to determine RHA revenue
targets with certain modifications dictated by the difference in scale. Fewer
age/sex bands would have to be used, but RAWP stated that this would result in
'insignificant' changes. On the other hand, RAWP was confident that
condition-specific (ie. ICD Chapter-specific) SMRs could continue to be used at
Area and District level. Although there would be some loss of reliability due
to smaller numbers, 'sensitivity tests indicate ... that the results will still
be closer to the notionally 'correct' result than would be the case if a cruder
measure, such as overall SMRs, were applied.' (DHSS, 1976c, p.40, para. 3.8.1).
Once again, the details of the actual sensitivity analysis were not included in
the report and the statement has to be taken on trust.

The quality of the argument for using SMRs in the RAWP formula given in the RAWP
final report has attracted considerable criticism. Soon after the report was
published the Radical Statistics Health Group characterised it as:

'This discussion of measures of need reads more as a post hoc justification
for the use of mortality statistics than as any genuine exploration of a
difficult problem.'
Radical Statistics Health Group, 1977, p.8)

Dearden (1985) commented on the very slender evidence advanced to support the use of SMRs, particularly sub-Regionally and the amount which has to be taken on trust. Yet despite the thinness of the evidence used to support the argument, RAWP's decision to employ SMRs has been extremely influential and survived a barrage of criticisms, perhaps because for the first time it enabled the use of factual evidence in place of political judgement to decide which parts of the country were in need of health care. The London Health Planning Consortium (LHPC), for example, following RAWP's lead, used SMRs in a fairly crude fashion in its method for defining strategic changes in acute bed numbers by specialty and District in London over a ten year period (London Health Planning Consortium, 1980). The LHPC took the projected population by age and sex for each District and determined an expected caseload in each specialty by applying projected hospitalisation rates to age-sex specialty groups. Adjustments were then made to take account of variations in morbidity and socio-environmental factors by multiplying the projected hospitalisation rates for each age-sex specialty group by the overall District SMR weighted for differential use between conditions in the District concerned. At about the same time the Advisory Group on Resource Allocation (AGRA), appointed by the Secretary of State for Social Services to consider detailed improvements in the RAWP methodology concluded on SMRs that, 'in the present state of knowledge no better method of allowing for morbidity in the RAWP formula is available' (DHSS, 1980b, p.25). AGRA advocated further research on the relationship of SMRs and social deprivation to demands on the NHS and the need for health care.

SMRs are still used in the national RAWP formula and in the majority of Regions, yet their inclusion, particularly in sub-Regional RAWP, has generated an extensive technical literature, mainly critical of their use. The main issues raised have been, the status of SMRs as proxies for morbidity measures; the relationship between SMRs and use of health services; the nature of the relationship between mortality, morbidity and need assumed in RAWP's use of SMRs; alternative mortality and morbidity measures for resource allocation; and the influence of social factors other than morbidity (eg. social deprivation) on need for health services. This literature is discussed in the remainder of this Chapter and in Chapter Five which follows it.

THE ADEQUACY OF MORTALITY DATA (SMRs) AS A PROXY FOR MORBIDITY

RAWP's use of SMRs has been extensively criticised as a poor measure of morbidity, but it is as well to remember at the outset that, 'since all measures [of morbidity] are contentious there is no simple way of resolving this continuing debate' (Bevan, Copeman, Perrin and Rosser, 1980, p.153). RAWP too was aware of the difficulty that, 'any allocation method based upon the data available may be open to challenge on grounds which will be difficult to either substantiate or refute' (DHSS, 1976c, p.11, para. 1.15). Nonetheless the Working Party was convinced that its data were sufficiently reliable to support the methods chosen. Others have been less certain that morbidity would mirror mortality. It is important to be clear that RAWP was using mortality data not as a proxy for overall population morbidity, but as a proxy for those aspects of morbidity (and thereby, the need for health care) which were known to vary geographically after the age/sex structure of populations had been accounted for.

Forster (1977) was critical of the analysis reported in the RAWP report comparing Regional SMRs with GHS morbidity data. The positive correlation between mortality and morbidity data, implying that the SMR was a good indicator of the need for health care was based on only one year's data with no account taken of possible sampling variation (DHSS 1976c, p.6, para. 2.9). Instead, in an influential piece of work which set the tone for much subsequent criticism of RAWP, Forster examined the correlation between age/sex standardised mortality rates and morbidity rates from the GHS for the 10 standard statistical regions for 1972 and 1973. He cast doubt on the relationship between mortality and morbidity. Rank order correlations between mortality and 'acute sickness' (restriction of normal activities because of illness/injury during a 2-week period before interview) and 'bed sickness' (acute sickness requiring a stay in bed during a 2-week period before interview) were not significant. However, there was a significant correlation between mortality and 'chronic sickness' (long-standing illness, disability or infirmity), but not between mortality and 'absence from work or school' (acute sickness necessitating time off work or school during a 2-week reference period). Forster (1977) concluded that mortality data might be a good proxy in developing countries where infectious disease is a major health problem and killer, but that the available evidence for England cast doubt on the validity of mortality data as an indicator of morbidity. Forster recommended that consideration should be given to removing SMRs from the RAWP revenue formula and suggested that GHS morbidity indicators might be useable instead, despite their acknowledged weaknesses. However, it is not clear from the article how this recommendation was justified particularly since GHS data are not available below Regional level. Forster's paper is often quoted as if it amounts to a definitive undermining of RAWP's choice of the SMR as a morbidity proxy. Yet the conclusions Forster drew from his results appear to be exaggerated. His results can be reinterpreted in support of RAWP's position. While 'acute', 'bed', and 'off-work' sickness were not found to be correlated with SMRs, these measures are likely to include episodes of illness which are not serious and which may not require any professional health service intervention. By contrast, 'chronic' sickness which was associated with mortality, would seem far more likely to include severe, long-standing illness and disability which would warrant extended use of health services. Chronic sickness is reponsible for far more use of NHS resources than acute sickness (Palmer, 1978). The argument about mortality and morbidity is complex and Forster's data do not amount to a case against the use of SMRs as a measure of the relative risk of needing health care.

Following Forster (1977), Snaith (1978) was also critical of RAWP's methodology for studying the correlation between mortality data and GHS self-reported 'acute' and 'chronic' illness and certified spells of incapacity at Regional level. Snaith queried the RAWP classification of Regions into "high", "medium" or "low" on mortality and morbidity measures. He showed that if the Regions are ranked according to mortality and then according to the various measures of illness, the level of agreement is much poorer than RAWP suggested (eg. Yorkshire and Humberside came top for morbidity but only fourth in mortality terms).

A third study at Regional level by Palmer (1978) used simple linear regression to test whether mortality measures were good indicators of morbidity and whether mortality measures were good indicators of the relative geographical risk of having a morbid condition. Palmer used a wide range of different morbidity measures including measures of utilisation (Hospital Inpatient Enquiry (HIPE) and GP consultation rates) infectious disease notifications, Cancer Registry data, GHS and ad hoc survey data. Many of the correlations with mortality data were equivocal, although there was some evidence that Regional patterns of mortality did mirror morbidity. Despite Regional mortality being a good predictor of variations in morbidity in statistical terms for certain diseases, especially cancers (eg. cancer of the stomach) and certain types of self-reported sickness (eg. chronic), Palmer was still critical of RAWP's decision to link SMRs to ICD code. This was because the need for health care was thus defined as the presence or absence of a pathological condition and impairment and disability were excluded from consideration. Palmer (1978) was critical of the crudeness of RAWP's use of SMRs by ICD Chapter headings since there was some evidence of greater variation within, than between, ICD Chapter SMRs in the association between mortality and morbidity. The association was far stronger in some Chapters than others, implying the need for an alternative classification of disease groups or the use of a small number of 'tracer' conditions as indicators of need. (Detailed studies of the relationship between service use and SMR <u>within</u> ICD Chapter are discussed below).

The inconclusive nature of this subject is shown by the fact that Forster (1978) carried out a similar exercise to Palmer (1978) and reviewed a range of available proxies for health care need (mortality data, notifications of infectious diseases, cancer registrations, hospital activity statistics, GP consultation data, health surveys and disability data). His conclusions remained far more critical of the use of SMRs. He concluded that mortality data were inadequate as a proxy for morbidity except for certain cancers. However it is unclear what he recommended in their place. Also it is questionable whether the theoretical limitations of mortality as an accurate measure of overall population morbidity apply with equal force to its use as a measure of the relative risk of needing health care, as in RAWP.

Despite the evidence of studies critical of the adequacy of the use of SMRs as surrogates for morbidity data, by no means all the research undertaken since 1976 points in the same direction. The case against the SMR as a proxy for morbidity remains at best, unproven. Indeed a number of recent studies lend emphatic support to RAWP's original choice of mortality data, in the absence of improvements in morbidity data. The principal studies are discussed briefly below. Brennan and Clare (1980) investigated the relationship between all-cause mortality in the age group 15-44 years, 45-64 years and over 65 years and two measures of morbidity from the 1971 national Census at County Borough level for the whole of England. The two measures of morbidity were 'sick and therefore unemployed' and 'permanently sick and therefore not seeking employment'. Both measures were regarded as indicators of morbidity towards the severe or urgent end of its spectrum. The authors recognised that the two measures did not cover the entire spectrum of morbidity. Strong linear relationships were obtained between mortality rates and morbidity rates. All the statistical relationships were highly statistically significant. Brennan and Clare (1980) concluded that mortality rates could justifably be used in RAWP as a proxy for morbidity and furthermore, at sub-Regional as well as Regional level. These results directly challenge Ferrer, Moore and Stevens' (1977), Forster's (1977) and Snaith's (1978) view that the association between mortality and mortality was doubtful sub-Regionally. The contrary results of Forster's 1977 study, for example, were put down to its very much smaller sample size by Brennan and Clare.

A number of other studies have demonstrated strong positive correlations between mortality and morbidity in most age groups even below District level. A recent study of the health experience of wards in Bristol has demonstrated a broad correspondence between four health indicators: SMRs for adults 15-64 years; combined stillbirth and infant mortality rate; mortality of adults over 65 years; and low birthweight (Townsend, Simpson and Tibbs, 1984). The degree of rank consistency of the 28 wards on the four indictors was high. In a similar piece of research, Townsend and colleagues studied three health variables (SMR 0-64 years, residents over 16 years 'permanently sick' at the Census and live births under 2800 grams) at ward level in the Northern Region. The SMR was found to be highly correlated with the other health variables (Townsend, Phillimore and Beattie, 1986). The Bristol and Northern Region studies show that mortality data cannot simply be rejected out of hand, particularly not before better morbidity data become available.

RELATIONSHIP OF MORTALITY TO SERVICE USE

Ferrer, Moore and Stevens (1977) noted that mortality statistics are unlikely adequately to reflect the variations in morbidity and service use preceding death from different conditions. Similarly many conditions are likely to generate a high use of services but not result in many deaths. In addition, their prevalence may not be closely correlated with their mortality rates (Fox, 1978, p.44). RAWP recommended SMRs calculated for broad groups of conditions in accordance with ICD Chapters for use in the formula for the non-psychiatric inpatient (NPIP) element of the revenue target. The SMRs were to be weighted by reference to existing national age/sex bed utilisation rates in addition to the age/sex structure of populations since it recognised the need to compensate for high mortality conditions leading to little health service use and vice-versa. Yet this procedure had the disadvantage according to the Radical Statistics Health Group (1977, p.9) and Lally (1980) of reintroducing historic supply-based weights and takes no account of policies such as the development of day surgery and provision for hip-replacements etc. which deal with disabling but not immediately life-threatening conditions (Royal Commission on the National Health Service, 1978b, p.12). Unfortunately, supply-based weights were all RAWP had available when it chose to make a partial adjustment to the influence of SMRs in the formula according to their contribution to bed use. Perhaps it would have been wiser to maintain the total "independence" of SMRs from existing patterns of supply. The main question for this discussion is, however, whether or not this method of weighting adequately adjusts condition-specific SMRs for differences in their associated service usage, particularly within the broad categories represented by ICD Chapters and in turn, whether this is a valid criticism of SMRs.

A range of studies have concentrated on the relationship between disease specific mortality (by ICD Chapter) and demand for hospital resources. ICD Chapters were designed to be homogeneous in terms of the nature of the diseases they comprise, not in terms of resource use. The Radical Statistics Health Group (RSHG) (1977) calculated the percentage of total deaths and bed use accounted for by each ICD Chapter in England in 1973. Three Chapters accounted for 85% of deaths and Chapter VII alone accounted for more than 50% of total deaths. Nine ICD Chapters accounted for less than 2% of deaths each, some less than 1%. As a result their SMRs were subject to considerable year-to-year fluctuation. For example, Chapter XII (diseases of the musculoskeletal system and connective tissue) accounted for less than 0.5% of annual deaths and as much as 6.8% of daily bed use in 1973. However, since RAWP was using mortality as a measure of relative not absolute morbidity, these facts do not necessarily invalidate the use of SMRs. Evidence of geographical variation in the prevalence of these diseases is required to support the RSHG criticism.

The complexity of the relationship between morbidity relevant to the requirement for health services and mortality was also highlighted by Walker (1978) who showed the lack of agreement at national level between deaths by ICD Chapter, and hospital admissions and the average number of beds used daily by ICD Chapter for 1973. Diagnoses of inpatients were spread over a far wider range of causes than deaths. Walker (1978) recommended more detailed comparisons between mortality and utilisation of individual diagnoses within ICD Chapters. These data draw attention to the fact that a large proportion of patients treated have conditions which are either unrelated to mortality (eg. hernia, varicose veins, cataracts, needs for care rather than cure, etc.) or conditions where any connection is coincidental or meaningless (eg. appendicitis). A national analysis of the average number of beds used by specialty, divided (as far as possible) into patients whose diagnoses were closely related to eventual cause of death and those not, revealed that probably half the occupied bed-days were used by patients whose diagnoses were not closely related to eventual cause of death (Walker, 1978). The author estimated that about three-quarters of general surgical inpatients suffered from conditions for which mortality is unconnected with the requirement for services and concluded that, 'the majority of inpatient hospital services are now predominantly of a rehabilitative, repair and caring type for which mortality data is inappropriate as an outcome measure' (Walker, 1978, p.6).

In response to this sort of analysis, it can be argued that:

1. While certain hospital death and discharge rates may reflect the incidence of disease, many do not and therefore, a lack of correlation between SMRs by ICD Chapter and deaths and discharges does not necessarily invalidate the use of SMRs as proxies for need.

2. Hospital utilisation rates in different disease categories reflect the importance attached in the past to identifying and treating different sorts of patients rather than an up-to-date reflection of community need for health services. Therefore one should not be too concerned about their lack of relationship with need indicators.

3. As long as the statistical relationship between hospital use (and other measures of morbidity, eg. from the GHS) and mortality is roughly constant across different Regions and Districts, mortality can be used as an indicator of relative need for resource allocation. Unfortunately, there appears to be relatively little analysis of this question within England. However, Bennett and Holland (1977) made the important observation, in defence of the use of SMRs in RAWP, that while deaths from common causes such as stroke, coronary heart disease and lung cancer tell us nothing about the prevalence of minor conditions such as hernia and varicose veins, there appears to be very little geographical variation except at small area level in the incidence and prevalence of these minor conditions. They also argue that the large majority of hospital admissions are generated by coronary heart disease, chronic bronchitis and related respiratory problems and that mortality is a good index of prevalence and therefore, of morbidity, for these. This is a helpful reminder of the fact that RAWP was using the SMR as a measure of relative geographical risk of need rather than as a measure of absolute morbidity.

4. RAWP chose mortality data specifically to have a measure of need independent of the supply and use of health services. It is therefore doubtful whether any evidence concerning the relationship between use levels and mortality rates is admissible in constructing the case against SMRs!

Geary (1977) carried out a more detailed exercise than Walker (1978) on mortality and service use, similar to that by the Radical Statistics Health Group (1977) reported above, but focusing on the sub-Regional level within Yorkshire RHA. Geary calculated SMRs for each ICD Chapter for the seventeen Districts in the Region. Chapters I (infective and parasitic disease), IV (blood and blood-forming organs), VI (nervous system), X (urinary system), XIII (musculoskeletal system and connective tissue), XV (perinatal mortality) and XVI (symptoms and ill-defined conditions), all led to high bed usage but few deaths. In each AHA these seven Chapters resulted in 28% of male and 25% of female bed use, but an average of only 300 deaths out of approximately 6000 annually in each AHA. Since the above Chapters accounted for few deaths, their SMRs fluctuated year-by-year at AHA and District levels to such an extent that for one AHA, a growth rate of +4% calculated using a two year SMR (1974-5) was turned into a rate of -0.7% by using the 1975 SMR alone. (The problems of fluctuations in SMRs sub-Regionally are discussed separately, below).

Geary's work highlighted the problematic status of the SMRs for a number of ICD Chapters, particularly the miscellaneous Chapter XVI (signs, symptoms and ill-defined conditions) which could be expected to exhibit an unusual pattern of mortality and resource use. Subsequently a number of suggestions have been made to improve the use of Chapter-specific SMRs in RAWP. In 1984 DHSS officials reviewed the use of Chapter XVI in national RAWP in a discussion paper for Regional Treasurers' consideration (DHSS, 1984a). Chapter XVI represented 0.4%

of deaths nationally, but 10% of national bed use on average. In such a case there was prima facie evidence that mortality was unlikely to be a good morbidity indicator. Furthermore, the proportion of beds occupied by patients with diagnoses within Chapter XVI varied from 3% to 20% between RHAs, further weakening the justification for its use in a formula directed towards Regional equity, since SMRs for Chapter XVI also varied between RHAs, but bore no relationship to Regional patterns of use.

Chapter XVI also demonstrated instability in both its SMR and bed usage from year-to-year. The small number of deaths in Chapter XVI even at Regional level meant that each death was assigned a higher than average weight in the calculation of the SMR and thus fluctuations in deaths could have a major unintended impact on RAWP targets. For example, when a single year's SMR data were used for target calculations in 1983-84, Northern RHA's target was reduced despite an increase in its overall SMRs, primarily because of a substantial drop in the male SMR for Chapter XVI. DHSS officials proposed using the all-cause SMR for Chapter XVI in place of the condition-specific SMRs for Chapter XVI in calculating targets, in order to reduce the impact of random variations in the attribution of deaths. This has now been accepted into the RAWP methodology and was used for the first time in the calculation of allocations and targets in 1985-86. DHSS officials regarded this as preferable to either setting the SMR at 100 or merging Chapter XVI with another Chapter. DHSS has considered whether other Chapters should be treated similarly, but concluded that Chapter XVI was unique in its combination of few deaths, high bed usage, Regional variations in death rates and bed usage and variation in Regional SMRs.

Similar problems with SMRs have led to setting the SMRs for ICD Chapter V (mental disorders), XII (skin diseases) and XVIII (persons without current complaint) at 100 for national RAWP purposes ignoring any possibly genuine Regional variations in death rates.

The Radical Statistics Health Group (RSHG) (1977) drew initial attention to the possibility that there might also be problems in the ICD Chapters encompassing large numbers of deaths, in that the SMRs of the constituent conditions within the Chapter might vary widely and account for a very different proportion of total bed usage. The RSHG reported that within Chapter VII, ischaemic heart disease and cardiovascular disease resulted respectively in 25% and 14% of the Chapter's deaths at national level, but different patterns of use of resources and mortality. A number of authors have looked at this issue in more detail.

West (1978) examined how closely mortality for England and Wales in a number of individual disease categories within ten Chapters of the ICD correlated with the demand placed by those categories on hospital beds using the Hospital Inpatient Enquiry (HIPE). West argued that since RAWP recommended that broad ICD Chapter SMRs be used in calculating the non-psychiatric inpatient (NPIP) revenue target, it was important to assess the homogeneity of ICD Chapters in terms of mortality and resource use. West (1978) found a significant level of correlation for disease categories within five ICD Chapters (neoplasms; diseases of the nervous system and sense organs; circulatory system; respiratory system; and muculoskeletal and connective tissue) and concluded that for these Chapters, use of the SMR in resource allocation was justified. However, West found a relatively poor correlation for diseases of the genitourinary system and the Chapter for accidents, poisoning and violence, indicating that for these Chapters the diseases making most demands on beds were not those making a major contribution to mortality. One possibility was to exclude such SMRs from the formula. An alternative was to calculate separate SMRs for each disease category within these ICD Chapters. West (1978) showed that within Chapter X (genitourinary disease) for females, genital conditions were responsible for 75% of the bed utilisation but less than 5% of the mortality. He concluded that it would be preferable in national RAWP to weight Regional populations by separate

national bed usage rates and separate Regional SMRs for this disease category
and also for male genital disease within Chapter X. He concluded that the SMR
for Chapter XVII (accidents, poisoning and violence) should be omitted
altogether. West's recommendations for change were aimed at RAWP distribution
to Regions, at which level SMRs for specific disease categories within ICD
Chapter could be be calculated with confidence. However, sub-Regionally with
smaller numbers of deaths this might be far less practicable.

Goldacre and Harris (1980) carried out an anlysis similar to Geary (1977) and
West (1978) to test the suitability of mortality data by ICD Chapter as proxies
for morbidity by studying the extent to which diseases which commonly result in
use of hospital care are also common causes of deaths within their ICD Chapter.
Rank correlations between deaths and hospital episodes (from HIPE) were
significant in 9 of 14 ICD Chapters and between deaths and beds used daily, in
12 of 14 Chapters. Inspection of the ranking of individual conditions showed
that most Chapters included diseases which were uncommon causes of death but
common reasons for hospital care. Chapters VI, VIII, X, XIII, XIV and XVI each
contained diseases which together accounted for less than 5% of the deaths in
each Chapter but more than 50% of the admissions in their Chapters. All
Chapters included a very wide range of conditions for which a single SMR was
calculated in the RAWP NPIP target. Most beds in ophthalmology, ENT,
gynaecology and dentistry and one third or more in general surgery, neurosurgery
and plastic surgery were used to treat conditions which were uncommon causes of
death, both absolutely and relative to their ICD Chapters. Goldacre and Harris
(1980) concluded that it was unlikely that the financial requirements for caring
for patients with these diseases could be adequately measured by employing
Chapter-specific SMRs in the RAWP formula. They recommended that if mortality
data were to be used in resource allocation, rates should be calculated for
diseases selected and grouped on the basis of research into the relationship
between mortality and the demands for care generated by diseases. Goldacre and
Harris also recommended that the grouping of conditions for resource allocation
purposes should match the grouping of services to be employed for planning;
whereas currently, hospital inpatient services are planned by specialty and care
group but funded according to a formula based on mortality data by ICD Chapter
and aggregated into a category of 'non-psychiatric in patient services' which is
unique to RAWP. (See Chapter Seven, 'Resource Allocation and Planning' for
further discussion of the need to reconcile the methods of resource allocation
and planning).

The relationship between mortality and the demand placed on services has also
been considered for different age groups. The Scottish Working Party on Revenue
Resource Allocation, for example, specifically excluded SMRs for the over-65s
from the Scottish formula (SHARE) on the basis that the need for health service
resources in this age group was determined by the elderly who survived rather
than those who died (Scottish Home and Health Department, 1977). It has been
argued that inpatient acute, day patient, ambulance services and community
health services should all exclude SMRs for the over-65s since they are
predominantly used by the old, the mentally ill and the mentally and physically
handicapped for whom there is probably an inverse relationship between "need"
and mortality (Varley, 1982, p.18).

Despite the number of studies demonstrating the poor correlation between deaths
and service use, the evidence they contain does not amount to a refutation of
RAWP's choice of mortality data. In defence of RAWP's original decision to use
SMRs as proxies for morbidity and need for services, Calum Paton adduces two
important arguments based on Bennett and Holland (1977) which may help place the
criticisms in context: firstly, that the main chronic conditions which exhibit a
poor correlation between prevalence and mortality, appear to show little
Regional variation; and secondly, that a large proportion of hospital admissions
are for coronary heart disease, chronic bronchitis and related respiratory

problems for which mortality is a good measure of prevalence and therefore of morbidity (Paton, 1985, pp. 59-60). However, the principal objection to studies such as Geary (1977), RSHG (1977), West (1978) and Goldacre and Harris (1980) is that they miss the point. Ultimately, the validity of SMRs as measures of need cannot be tested by examining relationships with what is provided since this does not indicate what is needed. RAWP was clear on this point. Subsequent critics were less so.

THE NATURE OF THE RELATIONSHIP BETWEEN MORTALITY AND NEED FOR RESOURCES

While researchers have questioned empirically the closeness of the statistical correlation between measures of mortality and a range of measures of morbidity with equivocal results (Forster, 1977; Forster, 1978; Snaith, 1978; and Palmer, 1978). The question still remains as to what a particular level of mortality (standing for morbidity) indicates in terms of the precise need for health care resources. Barr and Logan (1977) and Fox (1978) have questioned the simple assumption in the RAWP Report of a 1:1 relationship between mortality and need for health service resources (ie. that an SMR 10% above the national average indicates a requirement for 10% more in health resources). Can this easy assumption of linearity be sustained? It is known for instance that the availability of health services resources is not associated with noticeable reductions in mortality, since the majority of expenditure is on curative services. Changes in lifestyle and environment appear to have far more impact than health services in improving the health of populations, according to Barr and Logan (1977). Eyles, Smith and Woods (1982, p.241) were very critical of RAWP for pursuing a system for optimising the distribution of resources (and ultimately, services) with inadequate knowledge of the relevant input-output relations in the NHS. However, since the relationship between level of need, morbidity, inputs and outcomes is clearly complex, RAWP's assumption is difficult to justify or to refute. To depart from a linear assumption requires access to secure knowledge which is not available. In the circumstances the simplest assumption was probably inescapable. In a large-scale national study of the relationship between all-cause mortality and two morbidity measures from the Census at County Borough level, Brennan and Clare (1980) provide some evidence to support RAWP's assumption. The relationship between the two sets of variables was found to be broadly linear.

However, there have been criticisms not only of the nature of the relationship between morbidity, mortality and the need for health care, but also criticisms as to whether a high SMR necessarily indicates a high need for health care (Royal Commission on the National Health Service, 1978b, p.11). Critics argue that it would be preferable to use a definition of morbidity for resource allocation which relates directly to a need for health service resources rather than a need for other welfare services (Lally, 1980). A high SMR may indicate a need, but not necessarily for health care (eg. for better housing or a higher standard of living). RAWP was aware that expenditure on health services was not always the appropriate response to high levels of morbidity, but argued that although the impact of curative services might be marginal on morbidity (eg. for coronary heart disease), positive preventive measures and environmental changes could be promoted by health authorities (DHSS, 1976c, p.84, para. 6.32). Ashley and McLachlan (1985) go so far as to suggest that a high SMR may in fact be a measure of the _impotence_ of health services in an area to improve health and therefore, a measure of the need to invest in better housing, etc. rather than the NHS. RAWP attempted to overcome the criticism that the level of the SMR did not give a clear indication of the level of need for health services, by weighting ICD condition-specific SMRs by existing bed use rates. This reduced the weighting of the high SMR conditions with low bed use, but did so by reintroducing a supply-based element into resource allocation. Low bed use may be a historical reflection of the low priority assigned to meeting a particular need irrespective of the genuineness of that need.

Thus, a weakness of using either mortality or morbidity data as indicators of need for health care resources is the confusion as to whether these data are best used as "need" or "outcome" indicators. Forster (1978) argues that it is perverse to penalise a health authority financially when its SMR goes down, since this ignores the possible contribution of the effectiveness of its health services to this event. The health authority should be given some recognition for providing a good service. Others would be more sceptical of any close relationship between SMRs and effectiveness of health care delivery. Using mortality data alone it is impossible to distinguish between Districts with low SMRs because of low levels of morbidity or because of high levels of effectiveness. Sanderson (1979, p.20) posits the situation of two Districts with an equal incidence of a particular chronic disease, but in one District case fatality is lower than the other and so one District will have a higher prevalence with more people surviving to need caring for. The implication is that good medical care can alter the ratio between mortality and morbidity in certain circumstances. Thus by using mortality data alone, it is impossible to distinguish between DHAs with low levels of morbidity and those with high levels of effectiveness. However, RAWP was primarily concerned to secure equal opportunities of access to health care rather than equal efficiency or equal effectiveness. It would seem unreasonable to burden a single policy instrument with such intractable, multiple objectives. There is also the question of whether good medical care can make sufficient difference to mortality overall in a District to affect RAWP targets significantly.

ALTERNATIVE MEASURES OF MORTALITY

Weakness of the SMR as a Mortality Measure

Even if mortality data are deemed acceptable in resource allocation there is still the problem of deciding which indicator is most appropriate and feasible. Mortality indices (of which SMRs are perhaps the best known type) are all weighted averages of age-specific mortality ratios. As overall measures they do not reflect fully the mortality variations within different age/sex groups. However, the different indices vary in the weight given to each age/sex group based on the assumptions inherent in their method of calculation. SMRs are biased towards deaths in older age groups since the dominant role in determining the value of the SMR is played by the higher age-specific death rates (ie. in the age groups with the largest share of expected deaths) which, for most conditions, are to be found in the older age groups (Sanderson, 1979, p.16). Thus the SMR mainly reflects the relative mortality at older ages of an area compared with the national average. It is argued that this bias has two disadvantages in using SMRs as proxies for need for health services. Firstly, changes in age-specific death ratios at younger ages are more likely to reflect relative risks of needing health services than changes at older ages. In the elderly, chronic conditions generate a high demand for services but do not result in death and the mortality experience of individuals is likely to reflect the accumulated hazards of a lifetime rather than current circumstances. Secondly, the certified cause of death is less reliable at older ages and this will introduce a greater degree of uncertainty into the formula when the SMR is broken down by ICD Chapter (Palmer, West, Patrick and Glynn, 1979). The Scottish resource allocation formula (SHARE) eliminates SMRs for people over 64 years of age for these reasons (Scottish Home and Health Department, 1977), but Paton (1985) estimates that this procedure makes little difference to target calculations. Despite these drawbacks, the SMR is the only statistic available in cases where the local age-specific death rates are not known (Sanderson, 1979, p.14).

Barr and Logan (1977) criticised the validity of SMRs as a fair comparative measure of morbidity because all-age SMRs mask quite different death rates in different age groups. They quoted the fact that the Regional SMR for Oxford RHB in 1973 was 89 and for Newcastle, 115, but the death rate for the age group 5-24 years was lower in Newcastle than Oxford. After a comparison of mortality indices, Kilpatrick (1963) concluded that only when the age-specific mortality ratios (ASMRs) were not significantly different could the SMRs for different populations or areas be safely compared. Barr and Logan (1977) followed this advice and recommended that age-specific mortality ratios should be used in RAWP rather than SMRs where data were available. However, Sanderson (1979, p.14) went further and pointed out that it is even possible for populations with identical age-specific death rates to have quite different SMRs, since SMRs reflect not only death rates, but also the local population structure.

A further problem with the use of SMRs as recommended by RAWP was the decision to sum the estimates of bed usage for each age group and then to multiply this by an age-adjusted mortality index, the SMR. According to Sanderson (1979, p.23), it would have been better and more logical to estimate the age-specific bed usage, multiply by the age-specific mortality ratio and then sum. RAWP was against this on the grounds that the ASMRs for certain age group, condition and area combinations, would be based on small numbers of deaths and would therefore be unreliable. Sanderson (1979) rejects this argument. He argues that where low case fatality (eg. a chronic disease) is the reason for small numbers of deaths from a condition, mortality should not be used at all as an indicator of need and where rarity of the disease is the explanation for the small number of deaths, then instability in the ASMRs will have little impact on the final target. He concludes that ASMRs are preferable to SMRs where mortality is a good proxy for morbidity.

The Radical Statistics Health Group (1977, p.11) was critical of RAWP's lack of discussion of possible alternatives to SMRs for use in the RAWP formula and the absence of an explicit justification for choosing SMRs ahead of other possibilities. There was no indication in the Report of how different targets would have been using other measures. SMRs were probably selected because they were the best known and best understood mortality measure. However they may not have been the most appropriate conceptually.

The potential of other mortality measures for use in RAWP

Given that no index of mortality is independent of assumptions about the relative weight to be attached to deaths at different ages, the selection of a suitable indicator will always excite controversy. Palmer, West, Patrick and Glynn (1979) investigated the use of alternative mortality measures which might not be biased towards deaths in the older age groups as indicators of need in RAWP and their effects on targets. On conceptual grounds, the authors argued that age-specific mortality ratios (ASMRs), the relative mortality index (RMI) and Yerushalmy's mortality index (YMI) were more appropriate measures of the relative risk of dying than SMRs. The RMI was regarded as especially suited to a population-based method since it is the ratio of two populations. All three were stable, easily understood and easy to apply. The authors tested ASMRs, the RMI, YMI and the different approach of potential-years-of-life lost (PYLL) in the RAWP NPIP calculation and found that the formula was not robust with respect to the index of mortality used. If SMRs shifted the notional RAWP-weighted population from south to north, use of the other indices would accentuate this process, implying that SMR weighting leads to a 'minimum' level of redistribution. Northern, Yorkshire and North Western RHAs would gain consistently using ASMRs, RMI, YMI and PYLL. The effect of different mortality measures would be more marked below RHA level. Work in progress reported by Dearden (1985, p.10) which uses a similar methodology to Palmer et al (1979), suggests that changes from SMR-weighted targets at DHA level using various alternative mortality measures could be in the range from +20% to -15%.

However, such analyses do not tell us which index should be preferred if mortality data continue to be used in resource allocation. Although ASMRs, RMIs and YMIs are more suitable measures of relative risk of mortality on theoretical grounds, it cannot be assumed that they are better proxies for morbidity. According to Palmer et al (1979) this can only be decided by reference to the relevant health service policies, since use of any mortality measure involves assumptions about the relative importance of different age groups in weighting allocations (thus, YMI values an increased risk of death at any age equally, whereas the RMI and PYLL reverse the SMR weighting by emphasising deaths at younger ages). For example, it might be considered desirable to use an indicator which stressed relative change in death rates in younger age groups, since it is possible that greater provision for morbidity in the young and early middle-aged will prevent further illness and premature death. This sort of discussion of priorities raises the fundamental weakness in RAWP, explored in Chapter Seven, 'RAWP and Planning', namely the absence of adequate links between the process of financial allocation and forward service planning. In the absence of a deliberate mortality weighting by age based on an analysis of current policies and priorities, it has been recommended that the Age Specific Mortality Ratio (ASMR) is probably to be preferred to other measures of mortality, subject to adjustment for statistical significance (Holland, Charlton, Patrick and West, 1980). Sanderson (1979, p.23) similarly advocated the use of ASMRs in coordination with age-specific bed usage data for conditions in which there is a close association between morbidity and mortality and where the ASMRs are based on sufficient deaths to be stable.

ASMRs have received support as an attractive alternative to SMRs in more recent work. Pinder (1985) tested the technical properties of a range of measures and found that the Death Proportion Method, which is an all-age mortality index constructed from ASMRs, gave results indistinguishable from conventional SMRs when applied to the RAWP NPIP population but compared favourably in its standard errors. A further advantage of the Death Proportion Method was the fact that population data were not required in the calculations.

The published literature on mortality indices in RAWP focuses predominantly on the pros and cons of the SMR and other available summary measures since each measure inevitably makes approximations for specific mortality rates and assigns distinctive weights to deaths in different age groups. However, the possible use of crude death ratios with no age standardisation has also been discussed. Very soon after the RAWP report was published, Cochrane (1976) recommended that the RAWP formula should be simplified by replacing SMRs with crude death rates. Crude death rates for particular conditions could be applied to populations by sex and weighted by national utilisation patterns (Walker, 1978, p.8). It was argued that crude death rates without age standardisation were likely to give a closer approximation to the likely need for services than using age-standardised rates, at least in certain circumstances. This suggestion was not taken up by other writers.

Walker (1978) cites an example from Morris (1976, pp. 268-9) in support of the use of crude death rates. Morris argues that in a retirement town with a high proportion of elderly people in the population, the crude death rate is a more relevant indicator of the potential load on health services than the age-standardised rate. However, crude death rates share with SMRs, the drawback that they can only safely be compared between areas when the age-specific mortality ratios are not significantly different in the areas concerned. While Morris' point is valid in its own terms, it does not have a constructive bearing on the issue of comparative need which RAWP was trying to address. Cochrane's proposal to use crude death rates appears to rest on a misunderstanding. The crucial point is that RAWP was using SMRs not simply to account for morbidity differences (as many commentators have assumed in their criticism of the use of SMRs), but to overcome differences in morbidity between geographical areas which remain even when age and sex differences have been allowed for (ie. the SMR is a proxy for the relative risk of contracting a condition or needing health care in one area versus another) (Palmer, 1978). Much of the literature looks at the more general question of how accurately SMRs mirror morbidity variations, while it would be more relevant to ask the question: how good a measure of relative geographical risk of need is the SMR?

STABILITY OF SMRs AT SUB-REGIONAL LEVEL

The use of SMRs in RAWP was conceived primarily at the level of national RAWP targets for Regions. At Regional level, SMRs were found to be relatively stable from year-to-year (Geary, 1977). Analysis of the sensitivity of the national RAWP formula to the mortality data used in the calculation of targets indicated that RAWP was a robust method at Regional level since the Regional population dominated the target (Holland, Charlton, Patrick and West, 1980; Palmer, West and Dodd, 1980). The impact of statistically non-significant changes in SMRs (p>0.05) in the calculation of targets was small. Most RHA NPIP revenue targets changed by less than 1% when SMRs not significantly different from 100 (national average) were set to 100. From the evidence of this analysis, there was no indication that the use of SMRs was perverse at Regional level.

However, at sub-Regional level the use of SMRs has been extensively criticised. There are fewer deaths within each health authority at this level so that SMRs are likely to be less reliable and changes in SMRs tend to have a substantial impact on targets. Furthermore, there is considerable variation within Regions in the SMRs of different localities. The RAWP Report discussed possible changes in the population weighting in the formula for AHAs/Districts necessitated by the difference in scale, but concluded that ICD Chapter-specific SMRs could be used at this level and were preferable to overall SMRs, despite 'some loss of reliability due to the smaller numbers involved'. The Report continued:

> 'Sensitivity tests indicate, however, that the results will still be closer in most cases to the notionally 'correct' result than would be the case if a cruder measure, such as overall SMRs, were applied. As time goes by and the data base is built up from the 1 3/4 years used initially to the 10 recommended for eventual use, reliability will improve.'
> (DHSS, 1976c, p.40, para. 3.8.1).

The results of the sensitivity analysis were not reported making it difficult to challenge RAWP's enigmatic conclusion.

Geary (1977) calculated sex and Chapter-specific SMRs for the 17 Districts in Yorkshire RHA as recommended by RAWP. He showed random fluctuations in SMRs over time at this level due to the small numbers of deaths in each category. The SMRs gave a range of 225% about the RHA average in a single year. Fluctuations were such that in one District a growth rate of +4% calculated using two-year SMRs was converted into a rate of -0.7% by using one year's data alone (referred to above). A shift of +/-4% in the annual SMR for one ICD Chapter in one of the AHA's was worth about #1 million at 1977 prices. Geary was sceptical of RAWP's confidence that using ten-year SMRs would resolve the problem, since in his view ICD Chapters were inappropriate mortality divisions to use.

Snaith (1978) recognised, like Geary (1977), that at lower levels of aggregation the inadequacy of SMRs as criteria of need would become more marked. He was critical of RAWP's claim (quoted above) that ICD Chapter-specific SMRs should be used at this level in preference to overall SMRs. Snaith argued that the advantages of greater precision of more detailed SMRs would be cancelled by uncertainties because of the small numbers of deaths in each condition. However, according to Paton (1985) condition-aggregated SMRs theoretically have the drawback that as aggregate statistics they hinder a specialty by specialty attribution of utilisation and costs and thereby weaken the link with planning. Snaith concluded that SMRs were an inappropriate basis for deciding targets and allocations sub-Regionally.

In the early days of RAWP there were a number of other critical analyses of the frailties of SMRs sub-Regionally. Ferrer, Moore and Stevens (1977) found that the majority of District SMRs in the West Midlands RHA fell within their respective margins of random error when calculated from only one or two years' data. RAWP had advocated collecting up to ten years' data for use in SMR calculations to improve statistical reliability, but the authors were doubtful about using a cumulative sum technique to attempt to cancel random variation over a decade. The process would obscure important trends. Ferrer, Moore and Stevens (1977) concluded that there was a strong case for dispensing with SMRs below RHA level. Brennan and Clare (1980) reported the results for the West Midlands of calculating AHA revenue targets with and without SMRs. This produced variations in targets in the range from -3.7% to +5.9%. Commenting on these results, Bevan et al (1980, p.153) suggested that other morbidity measures might have been more appropriate sub-Regionally, since they could see little sense in using a surrogate estimate of need (ie. the SMR) if it yielded unstable targets. It would have been easier to cope with SMR fluctuations if RAWP had been able to justify abandoning the assumptions of a linear relation between SMRs and the need for resources.

Holland, Charlton, Patrick and West (1980) repeated their sensitivity analysis of the national RAWP formula using data from South East Thames RHA at AHA/District level in order to assess the reliability of ICD Chapter-specific SMRs sub-Regionally. At this level statistically significant variations in SMRs are more important and the NPIP target is more sensitive to SMR changes than at RHA level. The project team calculated that non-statistically significant SMRs accounted on average for approximately 2.5% of a District's NPIP target when three years of mortality data were used. The authors did not share Ferrer, Moore and Stevens' (1977) reservations about the use of SMRs based on 5-10 years' mortality data. They calculated that much of the instability in targets would disappear once an adequate run of data over time was available (Palmer, West and Dodd, 1980).

COPING WITH SMRs IN SUB-REGIONAL RAWP

A number of different ways of utilising SMRs in sub-Regional RAWP have been proposed in order to minimise the potential problem of instability and fluctuations in targets. Within the NHS itself a range of approaches have been adopted, including the use of alternative mortality measures as population weights (see above) and the replacement of mortality altogether by weights for morbidity or social deprivation (see below and Chapter Five). In the first few years of RAWP, a number of Regions simply omitted SMRs from the sub-Regional formula.

The most common approach was to replace ICD Chapter-specific SMRs with overall SMRs in the NPIP target (eg. Mersey RHA). West Midlands RHA opted to use condition-specific SMRs for only four ICD Chapters and overall SMRs in all other cases (NAHA, 1983). A joint Working Party of officials from DHSS and the Thames Regions recommended that for the NPIP target in London 'In sub-regional allocations, ... , we consider it preferable to use condition-aggregated SMRs to weight population' (DHSS and Thames Regional Health Authorities, 1979, p.5). This was primarily to overcome errors likely to arise because of small samples in sub-Regional condition-specific SMRs. Since 1979 certain Thames Regions have also introduced a variety of additional weightings to allow for differences in the social conditions prevailing in their Districts (see Chapter Five). The Joint Working Party also claimed that the use of aggregated SMRs helped to take some account of the problem of high bed use/low death rate conditions, since aggregated SMRs were essentially a summation of condition-specific SMRs for each AHA weighted to take account of national bed utilisation rates for each condition. For ambulance services' and community services' targets the Thames Regions used overall District SMRs (NAHA, 1983).

Academic commentators on RAWP have also produced suggestions for handling SMRs at AHA/District level. Geary (1977) was concerned to avoid large fluctuations in targets from year-to-year and proposed a range of possible responses:

1. ICD Chapters could be grouped together for the calculation of RAWP SMRs;

2. a single District/sex specific SMR could be used;

3. the RAWP formula could be restricted initially to a proportion of the NHS budget.

Geary (1977) did not discuss the fact that fluctuations in targets were only likely to be of great practical importance when Districts were approaching their targets and much less so at the beginning of the process of redistribution. In addition, there would appear to be no reason why actual allocations to health authorities should not be projected over a number of years, regardless of temporary fluctuations in SMRs, to enable managers to plan changes in services.

A convincing alternative approach to handling SMRs at AHA/District level is given by Holland, Charlton, Patrick and West (1980) (also in Palmer, West and Dodd, 1980). In the long-run, they advocated calculation of ICD Chapter-specific SMRs in the NPIP target using 5-10 years of mortality data when these became available. In the interim, their recommendation to Regions in calculating targets and allocations, was to use only those annual fluctuations in mortality which were statistically significant at the 5% level, to reduce the likelihood of large random swings in targets. Non-significant SMRs would be set at 100 for the calculation. The effect of this would be to reduce possible randomness in the NPIP formula at the expense of some degree of sensitivity in the process of allocation, since possibly "real", but non-significant SMRs would have been excluded. In South East Thames Region these SMRs accounted on average annually for about 2.5% of NPIP revenue targets. Holland et al (1980) surveyed Regional methods for using SMRs in sub-Regional RAWP and found that only two had taken detailed account of the statistical reliability of condition-specific SMRs for Districts.

USING MORBIDITY DATA IN PLACE OF MORTALITY DATA IN RESOURCE ALLOCATION

The logical extension of a critical analysis of the adequacy of mortality measures in RAWP is to consider whether it would be possible to use morbidity data similarly. Morbidity data have the disadvantages of being frequently less accurate than mortality data, far less comprehensive and more expensive to collect if they are to be independent of supply. In addition, they normally exhibit the same problem as mortality data, namely how to relate a specific level of morbidity to the need for a particular level and type of health care resources. In general, the data used for resource allocation should be as far as possible independent of the existing supply of facilities, but cover conditions and disease states which are either treatable or at least amenable to beneficial health service intervention. These two criteria are difficult, if not impossible, to reconcile.

Despite the fact that the available morbidity data rarely meet these criteria, a number of studies have assessed the feasibility of using existing morbidity data in resource allocation. Heasman (1979) excluded hospital statistics and identified three possible sources of available morbidity data, (sickness absence statistics, population surveys and GP morbidity statistics). He showed that the replacement of the SMR by an appropriate morbidity measure was 'not a short-term exercise'. Although population surveys similar to the GHS are an obvious development, Heasman showed that they would require very large sample sizes to produce statistically significant differences in health variables at sub-Regional level. The weaknesses of sickness absence statistics were well known. Existing GP morbidity systems would require extension to a properly representative sample of GPs before they could possibly be used in resource allocation.

Dajda (1979) developed a Regional morbidity indicator based on five self-reported, subjective, morbidity variables from the GHS in order to determine the proportion of resources which would be required by each Region to reach parity. When applied to Regional data for England and Wales, he found that the Regions lay on a continuum roughly corresponding to a south-east to north-west gradient of increasing morbidity which corresponded with a variety of indices of socio-economic conditions. Wales showed very different behaviour with a much higher reported morbidity, which could not be explained purely in socio-economic terms. Dajda (1979) recommended that further more detailed household surveys specifically directed towards health should be undertaken before using morbidity data in health service resource allocation, since the relationship between social conditions and self-reported morbidity was not constant between different constituent parts of England and Wales. RAWP had dismissed the self-reported morbidity data from the GHS because the national sample of only 15,000 households made it impossible to compile statistics below Regional level. Very large samples would be required to obtain District level data which could be used in RAWP.

RAWP was generally critical of morbidity data from surveys on the grounds that self-reported sickness was not a direct measure of the need for health care resources; differences in levels of reported sickness might be due in part to differences in perception and reporting of sickness; diagnostic categorisation would not be sufficiently reliable for resource allocation; the results of ad hoc surveys could not usually be extrapolated to national level; and adequate surveys at health authority level would be a difficult and costly business (DHSS, 1976 c, p.15, para. 2.7). In the time at its disposal RAWP could not have commissioned morbidity surveys, but its low opinion of their worth seems premature. There would seem to be a case for locally-based criteria of need derived from household surveys at District level (Curtis and Woods, 1984). The Black Report advocated such studies (DHSS, 1980a, p.215, para. 7.46). They could be developed in conjunction with other types of morbidity data such as disease registers.

Household surveys based on self-reported illness measures have only been infrequently carried out at District level. Almost without exception, resource allocation studies have used data collected for other purposes. There have been even fewer attempts to explore the links between health levels, service use and social factors in Great Britain using community morbidity surveys. However, two studies stand out; Skrimshire's survey of sickness in three areas (Skrimshire, 1978) and the 'Comparative Need for Health Care Project' (Curtis, 1983). This latter project aimed to measure and compare the prevalence of self-reported morbidity in two East London Boroughs with differing social characteristics (Tower Hamlets, typical of the inner East End and Redbridge, representing outer London) and to study the relationship between morbidity, demographic and socio-economic characteristics of respondents, and their use and perception of health services (Curtis, 1983). A random sample of 300 households in each Borough was interviewed using two main measures of morbidity, the 'long-standing and recently restricting illness' questions from the GHS and the self-completion, Nottingham Health Profile which measures perceived health problems and assesses the extent to which they affect activities of daily life (Hunt and McEwen, 1980).

Preliminary results showed a greater prevalence of morbidity in Tower Hamlets than Redbridge not explicable in terms of demographic factors and associated with a greater tendency to consult the GP. For example, 45% of Tower Hamlets adult respondents reported a long-standing illness (as defined by the GHS) versus only 35% in Redbridge. For acute sickness, overall prevalence in Tower Hamlets was 16% against 8% in Redbridge (Curtis and Woods, 1984). These results corresponded closely with the differential morbidity scores of respondents in inner and outer Manchester surveyed by the Department of General Practce, Manchester University using the same methods (Curtis and Woods, 1983). The London study indicated that socio-economic differences might account for some of the differences in morbidity. For some age groups, marital status, occupational class, housing tenure, educational attainment and ethnicity were associated with reported morbidity. These findings are of considerable interest since various of these social factors have been recommended for inclusion in the calculation of relative need indicators for resource allocation (Discussed in Chapter Five). Data on these variables are available from the Census for DHA populations throughout the country. However, since the impact of socio-economic variables was different in different age/sex groups and statistically significant in some but not others, the complexity of the interaction must be taken into account, if an attempt is to be made to link morbidity with social indicators for resource allocation purposes. Furthermore, as far as RAWP methods are concerned, what matters is whether the morbidity variations observed between Tower Hamlets and Redbridge are similarly observed for mortality. If they are, then this supports the continued use of mortality data as a morbidity proxy in sub-Regional RAWP. Unfortunately, these correlations were not reported in Curtis (1983). The implications of the 'Comparative Need for Health Care Project' are discussed below.

The second morbidity study relevant to RAWP was a small-scale, comparative, pilot study of the health experience of people in three socially homogeneous but distinct areas: a new working class council estate in socially deprived Newham (well above national average SMRs); a "problem" working class estate in a prosperous part of the Midlands (below average SMRs); and a prosperous middle class owner-occupied district in the same part of the Midlands (below average SMRs) (Skrimshire, 1978). In general, the self-reported morbidity of the samples matched what one would have predicted from the mortality rates prevailing in the localities (ie. Newham with much higher mortality rates especially in the elderly) and distinguished sharply between Newham with above the national average rates of morbidity and the then-prosperous Midlands with below average rates. This would tend to support RAWP's decision to use SMRs as a morbidity proxy. However, the Newham sample reported especially high rates of chronic sickness among children, particularly respiratory symptoms which were not predictable from its mortality experience. There was some evidence that sickness rates in children were worse in a deprived area (Newham council estate) than in a non-deprived area (Midlands council estate) whose population contained a similar working class population. This draws attention, for example, to possible environmental hazards in the neighbourhood which may not be adequately reflected in either an indicator of the social class composition of the population or in its mortality rates. Skrimshire's case studies would tend to indicate that in the absence of detailed morbidity data it may be necessary to include measures of social and environmental deprivation in the process for assessing the need for health care in resource allocation. However, it would be preferable to institute a series of similar morbidity surveys across the country for resource allocation purposes rather than relying on social indicators as proxies for morbidity. Furthermore Skrimshire's study was of three small areas well below the size of the health Districts used in RAWP. It is unlikely that the variations in the morbidity:mortality relationship which she describes would show up at the level of a District RAWP target. The issue of whether there should be an allowance for social and environmental conditions in RAWP is covered in the next Chapter.

Health care professionals tend to express scepticism not so much at the feasibility and expense of health interview surveys, but about whether or not they measure variations in health and well-being which can or should be responded to by formal health services. There is always likely to be a contrast between professional norms and perceived needs reported by members of the public. For example, it can be argued that household surveys will detect minor conditions which may not be indicative of the need for health care, particularly not hospital care. It is further argued that the results may be more an expression of respondents' expectations than their objective health status. One or two experimental projects have tried to combine the health interview survey with professional definitions of need, either by using a panel of doctors to transform data into normatively-determined need for health care expressed in terms of hospitalisation, tests, visits, etc., or by supplementing patient-reported symptoms with simple objective data or even physical examinations of respondents (Ashley and McLachlan, 1985, pp. 56-57). These elaborations of the community survey tend to be laborious and expensive and presume the inferiority of self-reported morbidity data without necessarily exploring the advantages which such data can afford.

What are the implications for resource allocation policy of comparative surveys such as the Tower Hamlets/Redbridge Study (Curtis, 1983; Curtis and Woods, 1984)? The results suggest a higher prevalence of self-reported illness in the inner city compared with outer London and the population of Great Britain in general. Yet since this broadly matches what would have been expected from the mortality experience of the same areas, the question arises as to whether morbidity data from surveys possess any additional properties which would justify their use in resource allocation. Once again RAWP's choice of mortality is shown to be basically sound for hospital and community health services. However, the proponents of community surveys see the principal advantages of self-reported morbidity data over other measures for resource allocation as follows:

1. Self-reported morbidity data are likely to correspond more closely to health-related attitudes and behaviour and respondents' propensity to improve or maintain their health. This feature may be especially relevant to planning health promotion and preventive services.

2. Self-reported morbidity measures may be particularly valuable in measuring the need for health services generated by non life-threatening disease, chronic illness, disability, or stress-related complaints which can have a serious impact on quality of life, but for which mortality statistics may be an inappropriate proxy (although evidence suggests that mortality data are not such poor indicators as is commonly imagined). These conditions may have considerable signficance in terms of resources, particularly for primary and community health services or outpatient hospital services.

3. Self-reported morbidity data comprise lay definitions of need and therefore have the potential to contribute to a resource allocation policy which reflects not only professional views, but wider societal judgements about how health care resources should be distributed (Curtis and Woods, 1983).

Curtis and Woods thus view community morbidity data as a way of enhancing conventional need indicators, particularly for primary and community health services, caring services for the disabled and chronically ill and health promotion and preventive services. Morbidity data from community surveys are regarded as most appropriate for these services because these are services designed to be delivered to geographically-defined populations from which survey samples can be drawn. It would seem theoretically possible to use self-reported morbidity data in combination with conventional indicators (eg. mortality data and clinical definitions of need) to enhance these more familiar measures for geographical resource allocation of community health services etc. in RAWP. The link between self-reported morbidity and other surrogate indicators of need (eg. housing tenure, social class composition of the population, etc.) could also be exploited so that the relative need assessments from community morbidity surveys in a sample of Districts with differing socio-economic characteristics could be generalised to all Districts using Census data. The important step is to validate the social indicators by reference to surveys independent of the supply of resources.

If the approach piloted by Curtis and Woods (1983) is to be applied routinely to resource allocation in the Health Service, finance will be required for a coordinated programme of District health surveys to map spatial variations in community health, independent of service use and to complement mortality data. Regular surveys near to the date of the national Census would be particularly useful because they would enable a check to be made on the representativenss of samples and an exploration of the statistical relationship between morbidity and social factors. However, Curtis and Woods also see the need for more frequent surveys between times, to gauge changing needs. Compared with the use of the SMR or other routinely available proxies for need, the population survey approach is expensive. This is a drawback in the NHS which lacks a firm tradition of investing in research and development. There is reluctance to change this, particularly when the NHS is in the throes of developing new routine computerised information systems which are thus in competition for funds with the requirements of research. Hitherto, the RAWP procedure at national level has relied entirely on easily available data collected routinely for other purposes. Yet in terms of the scale of financial resources to be reallocated through the RAWP procedure, an investment in surveys may be seen as no more than prudent planning.

Morbidity data generated routinely within the NHS have also been considered for possible use in resource allocation. Gandy (1979a) explored the suitability of substituting the standardised notification rate (SNR) for the SMR for respiratory tuberculosis in the RAWP formula, since the SMR lacked consistency from year-to-year because of the small number of tuberculosis deaths. Gandy (1979a) correlated SMRs and SNRs by sex for the 14 former RHBs and Wales with the discharge rate for respiratory TB from HIPE. The SNR was more sensitive to the presence of Asian population morbidity which increases the demand for services in certain parts of the country (eg. Leicester). He concluded that the SNR was a better proxy for morbidity in respiratory TB and probably in other infectious diseases, than the SMR. He recommended that since it was unlikely that a universal proxy measure of morbidity could be found, the aim should be to identify the best proxy measure for each group of diagnoses from a range of sources. For example, National Cancer Registry data might be more appropriate for cancers than mortality data.

In a recent conference paper Baker and Kernohan (1985) argue a similar case for the use of morbidity (prevalance) data in weighting the mental handicap component of RAWP targets in cities with large Asian populations. Yorkshire RHA calculates District targets for mental handicap using a modified RAWP method which includes an allowance for the location of long-stay mental handicap patients. This enables DHAs to fund community care for patients transferred from the long-stay hospitals, but takes no account of provision for new cases which have never been hospitalised. Bradford District has a higher prevalance of mental handicap associated with the presence of a large Asian population from Pakistan with an incidence of mental handicap approximately three times the white population. Such a District is disadvantaged in RAWP since these cases are all children who have never been hospitalised, in conformity with current thinking and who therefore, attract no funds. Consequently, Baker and Kernohan recommend that age/sex structure, numbers of long-stay patients and prevalence should form the basis of adjustments to RAWP targets for mental handicap in Bradford and all other cities with a large Asian population. This may not be a problem except in Yorkshire RHA, since many Regions have removed mental handicap from RAWP altogether and fund mental handicap developments separately. A similar case could be made for mental illness services. There is evidence to suggest that the prevalence of mental illness is higher in Regions with large conurbations (eg. London, Manchester and Birmingham) and that this should be incorporated in RAWP.

Overall, the use of morbidity data has not found favour with Regions for use in sub-Regional RAWP. Few are able to spend the money which would be needed for community morbidity surveys and little attention has been paid to extending existing, routine systems such as cancer registrations to other conditions. In the absence of agreed measures of relative need, attention has focused on social indicators as proxies for health service need, (ie. the extent to which the social characteristics of an area are associated with the demand and need for health services prevailing in the area). This sort of analysis has become inextricably linked with the political debate about whether relatively high spending, socially deprived, inner city Districts should be obliged by RAWP to surrender resources to less well provided but less socially deprived Districts, in the name of equity. The "social deprivation and resource allocation debate" is covered in the next Chapter. One attraction of using social indicators rather than mortality or morbidity data to make allocative decisions is that it eliminates the confusion engendered by employing the same data to measure need as outcome. Forster (1978) made one of the earliest proposals for including social indicators in the RAWP formula instead of mortality or morbidity data. He suggested using the social class composition of the population as a possible crude indicator of need, not only because of the well-known association between social class and morbidity, but also because health service activity in itself is most unlikely to affect the social class composition of a locality. Under this proposal, for example, a health authority would not be financially penalised for reducing its mortality and morbidity rates through a health promotion strategy. On the other hand, an authority which chose to put greater emphasis on curative and caring services with no visible impact on SMRs would equally not be at a disadvantage.

The focus on applying social indicators to RAWP has tended to detract from the potential contribution of a variety of measures of mortality and morbidity to estimating the health care needs of a District. This is unfortunate since better morbidity data could play an important part in future methods of resource allocation sub-Regionally. Ashley and McLachlan (1985) suggest a varied approach in which for a limited range of diseases with very high case fatality rates (eg. selected cancers and acute myocardial infarction), SMRs (or ASMRs) could be used as indicators of morbidity for the purpose of achieving equity in the distribution of resources. The assumption would be that for these diseases morbidity and mortality are causally linked. These mortality data could be complemented by a series of local case registers for conditions such as ischaemic heart disease, stroke, mental handicap, etc., where there is a suspicion that mortality may not be such a good indicator of need. These registers could be based on an extension of existing registers, using record linkage and standard criteria. The choice would be to include rarely fatal, but burdensome, chronic conditions which are known to contribute to the overall needs of a community for a range of health services. However, disease registers are costly to maintain and unfortunately, appear best suited to those diseases for which mortality data are a suitable proxy.

There is also undeniably potential for collecting data from population morbidity surveys. These have the great merit of providing data reasonably independent of the supply of health service facilities. However, these pose a variety of problems, particularly how to quantify the needs for specific types of health care (eg. inpatient, day patient, community support, GP care, etc.) from subjective assessments of self-reported sickness. However, the basic epidemiology required for an objective method of resource allocation based on morbidity now needs to be undertaken. Although mortality data are the best source we currently have, RAWP's epidemiological approach should be continued so as to establish basic measures of need from morbidity studies. It will be particularly important for geographical resource allocation to have a better understanding of whether there is any major spatial variation in the prevalence of the chronic conditions where mortality and morbidity are not likely to be causally linked. The available evidence suggests that there is little systematic geographical variation in those chronic conditions for which mortality is a poor proxy of prevalence, but this evidence requires updating and expanding (Bennett and Holland, 1977).

The collection of morbidity data through community surveys will be expensive, but it should be possible to carry out such studies in a representative cross-section of Districts which would enable the results to be generalised (within limits) to Districts with similar population or environmental characteristics. This would maximise the value of these studies.

CONCLUSIONS

RAWP's use of SMRs as a measure of relative morbidity has been extensively criticised since 1976, yet in the intervening years there have been few if any improvements in the quality or coverage of routine morbidity data collected in the NHS (Ashley and McLachlan, 1985). RAWP's choice of mortality data was constrained by the fact that there was no other morbidity proxy which was independent of the existing supply of health service resources, accurate, reliable, comprehensive, available regularly by Region and District and able to be broken down by age, sex and diagnosis. The same is still true. Virtually no progress has been made since 1976 to provide better routine need data than mortality.

Studies which have looked at the correlation between mortality and morbidity indicators have as often as not supported the original analysis presented to RAWP, which showed the high geographic correlation of SMRs with a range of available morbidity statistics. Despite this, an orthodoxy has developed in the NHS that SMRs are inappropriate in RAWP. While SMRs may not be an equally good surrogate for morbidity in all conditions and for all age groups, the evidence does not amount to a case for dropping mortality from RAWP. Forster's analysis of the correlation between General Household Survey (GHS) sickness data and SMRs has been influential and is often quoted to show that SMRs cannot be used in RAWP to measure morbidity (Forster, 1977). Yet a closer inspection of the results shows the complexities of the argument. Forster showed a statistically significant correlation between GHS chronic sickness and SMRs at Regional level, but not a significant correlation for acute sickness or bed sickness or sickness causing work or school absence. He concluded that it was doubtful if mortality could be considered a valid indicator of morbidity. However, Forster's conclusion appears perverse when it is recalled that RAWP was using the SMR not as a measure of global morbidity, but as a measure of the relative risk of needing health care. Acute and off-work sickness which were not correlated with SMRs will include episodes which are not life-threatening and which may not require any health service intervention. By contrast, chronic sickness which was correlated with SMRs would seem much more likely to include severe, long-standing illnesses and disabilities which would warrant health service help. Chronic sickness is known to account for far more resource utilisation in the NHS than acute sickness (Palmer, 1978). Ferrer, Moore and Stevens (1977) and Snaith (1978) followed Forster in arguing that the level of correlation between mortality and morbidity was even poorer, below Regional level; but again without considering the extent to which the morbidity measures they used were, or were not, likely to reflect the need for health care. In fact there have been at least as many, if not more, studies whose conclusions point in favour of the use of mortality data in RAWP, in the absence of good direct measures of morbidity. Brennan and Clare (1980) for example, in a much larger study than Forster's (1977), analysed the statistical relationship between mortality and two measures of sickness from the national Census and found strong correlations even below the level of the former Area Health Authorities. Although the two Census morbidity measures were not ideal, they were measures towards the severe or urgent end of the morbidity spectrum likely to require professional help. Brennan and Clare (1980) concluded that mortality data could justifiably be used even sub-Regionally as a proxy for morbidity in resource allocation. It would seem therefore, that the case against the use of mortality data in RAWP remains unproven on grounds of the relationship between mortality and morbidity.

The second principal criticism of the SMR has been on the grounds that many conditions are likely to generate a high use of services but not result in many deaths and vice-versa (Radical Statistics Health Group, 1977; Goldacre, 1981). It is argued that mortality statistics are unlikely to reflect variations in morbidity and service use preceding death from associated but different conditions. Studies showing the discrepancies between conditions accounting for deaths and those leading to service use appear damning, but carry little weight. Firstly, there is little evidence to suggest that the relationship between mortality and service use varies significantly between different parts of the country. RAWP was after all, using the SMR as a measure of relative geographical risk of need (Bennett and Holland, 1977). Secondly, these criticisms rely on statistics of health service use which RAWP explicitly refused to take into account, for the simple reason that such statistics do not indicate the need for health care as much as the availability of facilities in particular areas. It seems perverse to criticise RAWP for choosing a surrogate for need which was "independent" of supply on the grounds that it actually was "independent" of supply! To invalidate SMRs by their lack of relationship with the utilisation patterns generated by current health services, assumes that current services are optimally arranged to meet (and therefore, reflect) health needs in the population. This seems highly unlikely. However, to be entirely consistent in rejecting data on use of services, RAWP should perhaps have avoided weighting the population by reference to national utilisation rates in each ICD Chapter.

The discussion of alternative morbidity measures which could be used in place of SMRs underlines a general difficulty for critics of the SMR if they wish to be constructive rather than merely destructive: what are they to put in its place? Critics tend to be coy of suggesting alternatives. The available morbidity measures all require substantial investment before they could be used in RAWP. The best quality sources tend to cover only a few conditions and/or are restricted to particular areas. None are as comprehensive as mortality data. Each tends to identify a particular facet of the complex phenomenon of "morbidity". Many are known to be inaccurate (Ashley and McLachlan, 1985).

Faced with the cost of collecting morbidity data themselves or finding a cheaper and easier option, a number of Regional Health Authorities have begun to explore the potential of widely available social indicators for use in RAWP in place of SMRs. In the main, this has been a Regional response to criticisms that SMRs not only fail to account adequately for morbidity, but furthermore, that they underestimate the needs of socially deprived areas, especially in the inner cities. Adverse social factors are said to place extra burdens on health services or make a given level of provision more difficult to accomplish for any given level of morbidity (Fox, 1978; Woods, 1982). The first response to RAWP's choice of the SMR after 1976 was to criticise mortality data as proxies for morbidity per se. However, latterly critical attention has shifted to consider whether mortality can adequately encapsulate not only need expressed in the form of morbidity, but additionally, need in the form of the social conditions in which people live their lives. The next Chapter attempts to assess the justification for this extension of the original case against SMRs.

CHAPTER FIVE

SOCIAL DEPRIVATION AND THE NEED FOR HEALTH CARE

THE "RAWP AND SOCIAL DEPRIVATION DEBATE"

The importance of socio-economic factors as determinants of health, perceptions of health, health-related behaviour, use of health services and therefore, of the need for health services, is well recognised. However, RAWP chose to make no separate allowance for the effect of socio-economic conditions on either the health of populations and their health care needs, or on the circumstances in which health care is provided. RAWP was aware that there was considerable evidence of strong associations between a wide range of population socio-economic characteristics (eg. social class) and the demand for health care. However, RAWP assumed that social conditions in an area would be reflected in local mortality experience and that including an allowance for additional social factors besides mortality would run the risk of 'double counting'. Furthermore, RAWP argued that:

> 'Health programmes are not the only means of improving health in a locality. We recognise the important influences of other factors, eg. housing, environmental health facilities, working conditions etc. Except in the sense that they all have an impact on the morbidity of populations, we cannot take them into account. They are the province of other social programmes and the extent to which they react with the health care programme is not an issue with which we are equipped to deal.'
> (DHSS, 1976c, p.11, para. 1.16)

RAWP was clear that tackling the problem of social deprivation was not primarily the responsibility of the NHS and certainly not the responsibility of the resource allocation mechanism. Other agencies were in a better position to effect improvements in wider socio-economic conditions. It seemed reasonable to suppose that social deprivation would result in an increased susceptibility to disease and death which would show up in mortality figures; although it would seem likely that recent mortality rates were a product of past rather than present social circumstances. However, there is bound to be a lag between changes in socio-economic conditions and their effect on the need for health care.

The adequacy of RAWP's stand on social deprivation has been the subject of extensive debate, most of it criticising the lack of a "social deprivation weight" in sub-Regional RAWP which would take account of the effect of adverse social conditions over and above those which are visible in mortality (Lally, 1980). The social deprivation question has been treated as a predominantly sub-Regional issue since, although not all RHAs exhibit the same levels of social deprivation, the scale of variation between them is substantially smaller than between inner city, suburban and rural districts within Regions. In a number of Regions, changes have been made in the methods of sub-Regional resorce allocation in an attempt to reflect a wider definition of "need" than morbidity. On the other hand, RAWP was concerned primarily with devising a formula for allocations by DHSS to Regions, so it is understandable that the issue of social deprivation was not discussed in depth. It is now virtually an NHS orthodoxy to criticise RAWP for not including an allowance for social deprivation. This Chapter attempts to look at the evidence which would support this view and to appraise the steps which have been taken by Regions to remedy the "incompleteness" of mortality data in RAWP. The literature and discussion of area variations in deprivation and health in the NHS have generally failed to clarify what is meant by "social deprivation" in the context of NHS resource allocation and the need for health care. Measures based on the characteristics of areas and of individuals and measures combining both sorts of variable, have been used interchangeably. Measures of social status have also been put forward as alternatives to SMRs in the guise of measuring social deprivation. The tendency has been to select social variables in an arbitrary fashion without adequate consideration of their theoretical relevance to the need for health care.

Many have taken the view, for a variety of theoretical and expedient reasons, that SMRs are 'an incomplete proxy for need because they do not recognise urban poverty, crowding and other effects of social deprivation' (Fox, 1978, p.44). There are thus two main strands to the argument about social deprivation and need for health service resources:

1. firstly, that social deprivation results in a higher level of need for health care in clinical terms than mortality rates would lead one to expect (ie. in socially deprived areas, the ratio of mortality to morbidity is different than in non-socially deprived areas);

2. secondly, that adverse social factors place extra demands on the NHS for any given level of clinical morbidity which it is unlikely that SMRs can adequately take account of. The argument is that the relationship between morbidity and the need for health care resources varies depending on the socio-economic and environmental characteristics of an area. For example, hospitals in deprived areas may be obliged to compensate for inadequacies in housing conditions of patients through longer lengths of stay or lower admission thresholds (Royal Commission on the National Health Service, 1978b, p.12; Woods, 1982, p.76). It has also been claimed that deprived people may find it more difficult to cope with minor illness and to use health services appropriately than the non-deprived, leading to low up-take of services and the necessity for "outreach" programmes and other special provision requiring extra expenditure by health authorities (Lally, 1980, p.34).

This second strand in the argument would defend the right of the NHS to compensate for social conditions and inadequacies in other welfare services, on the grounds that it already does so every day in normal clinical practice. This begs two questions: is this an accurate description of what really occurs in hospitals in deprived areas; and is the NHS the most cost-effective agency to perform this task?

RAWP's decision not to include deprivation resulted not only from its members' interpretation of the limits of their remit, but also from unpublished, DHSS research evidence presented to the Working Party which showed that in geographic terms, SMRs were highly correlated with a number of indicators associated with social deprivation and lower social class areas (ie. poverty, the proportion of unskilled manual workers, early termination of education, unemployment, public housing, large families and lack of higher education) (DHSS, 1976d). These indicators tended to have high values in northern Metropolitan Districts. As a result of this analysis RAWP felt justified in not making extra allowance for adverse social conditions and concluded that they were, for practical purposes, mirrored in raised SMRs.

However, these DHSS data were not uniformly consistent and were open to interpretation. Buxton and Klein remind us that RAWP had available further data from the same DHSS report which showed that there was no geographical association between SMRs and some of the indicators which (in their view) tended to be associated with "problem areas" [sic] in Inner London rather than in cities in the North of England. These were variables such as the proportion of immigrants in the population and the proportion of people in private rented accommodation (Royal Commission on the NHS, 1978b, p.12). The implication seemed to be that RAWP was biased against London and its morbidity indicators might be peculiarly inadequate in London with its unique blend of social deprivation (Lally, 1980). Accordingly, Buxton and Klein ask whether RAWP should take account of social conditions which are not necessarily reflected in mrobidity, but affect demand for services. The indicators of "problem areas" (it is not clear what a "problem area" comprised!) they had selected tended to be social rather than material or economic factors. It was possible that the inconclusive nature of the data on the relationship of SMRs and deprivation was the product of differing interpretations of what constituted "deprivation".

Academic critics were joined by those who had to deliver curative and caring services in socially deprived areas. Staff had misgivings about whether mortality data could ever adequately describe the conditions they faced. To what extent and in which ways was their work made more difficult or costly by social conditions? To what extent did other features of socially deprived areas and behavioural characteristics of their residents place a greater than expected burden on the NHS? These are difficult questions to answer objectively, but in the immediate aftermath of the publication of the RAWP report clinicians (it must be said, almost exclusively from inner London teaching hospitals) fired a volley of articles and correspondence at the heads of members of the Working Party, rebuking their naivety in not including a social deprivation weighting in RAWP. The coincidence of commonsense observations from their own practice (eg. that discharges might be delayed because of poor home conditions) and the realisation that the most over-target AHAs tended to be in deprived inner city areas, particularly in London, made them sure that SMRs were inadequate. The "social deprivation debate" was initiated in the medical press by Sir Francis Avery-Jones of the Middlesex Hopital who put the case for the hospitals serving poor areas in inner London forcibly and eloquently, but with scant attention to the few facts which were established. The main impetus to his contribution appeared to be the fact that London faced a standstill in resource growth as a result of RAWP. At bottom he was hostile to the very idea of allocating health service resources on the basis of need rather than use, but chose the absence of an allowance for inner city factors as the main thrust of his criticism of RAWP. He argued that expenditure in London was high not because of extravagance and higher standards of care, but because of 'conurbation factors' such as overcrowding, unemployment, population morbidity, pollution, the proportion of elderly people living alone, etc...' Unplanned, historical accident was conveniently overlooked! '... It is much more expensive in terms of beds and staff to provide medical and social services for a deprived area than for an affluent one', he asserted (Avery-Jones, 1976, p.1047). He claimed that if metropolitan market cost factors and social deprivation were taken into account the spending of the Thames RHAs would not be found to be excessive. He regarded it as illogical that a healthier, less deprived Region like East Anglia with cheap to provide, efficient services should gain through RAWP ahead of London with worse SMRs and greater social deprivation. He chose to ignore the main reason for the relative position of the two Regions under RAWP, which was the marked difference in levels of expenditure per capita. While he recognised that the long-term solution to social deprivation was to improve the social environment, Avery-Jones recommended in the short term that 'Additional resources and more hospital beds are needed to meet the greater medico-social needs of such areas' and urged the Government to reconsider RAWP.

Avery-Jones' critique was taken up by Whimster (1976) who argued that RAWP's aggregate approach was a crude administrative solution to the complex problem of taking into account social class structure and deprivation in resource allocation and reflected the non-clinical nature of the Working Party. The British Medical Journal supported the clinicians' case with a leader entitled 'What a RAWP roar' (Anonymous, 1976b), pointing out that since 'to some extent at least medical services have become concentrated in areas of high morbidity' RAWP was overstating the need for reallocation. The leader was also critical of the use of SMRs and the rejection of factors relevant to need such as population density, occupational structure, poverty, lack of knowledge and social class composition of localities (precisely how these were relevant and were to be measured was not stated).

The medically qualified members of the Working Party and its sub-committees replied to their clinical colleagues' criticisms (Forsythe, Holland, Lane, Bennett and Snaith, 1976). RAWP's remit had been limited to the Health Service and they did not believe that it should be the function of the NHS to remedy the inadequacies of social services, housing, employment, etc. This would lead to wasteful palliatives while ignoring the causes of deprivation. They admitted that the RAWP Report had recognised that deficiencies in housing and social services 'impose an added burden in certain places which cannot be ignored in the short term' but had not put forward any specific proposals for responding to this problem. However, they reminded critics that the Report had stressed that the pace of movement towards 'targets' would be at the discretion of Ministers and RHAs and that it would be possible to take account of local factors if necessary, through this process. The Report stated:

'Authorities will also need to bear in mind the real but unquantifiable impact upon the services they provide of deprivation in a wider social sense. It is conceivable that a particular AHA or District would always be maintained at a level above its indicated target. (DHSS 1976c, p.41, para 3.9)

What RAWP was anxious to avoid, however, was a situation in which deficiencies in housing, working conditions, social services, etc. would be built into the long-term assessment of a health authority's relative need for funds, thus introducing or retaining permanent distortions in the local pattern of health services.

Buxton and Klein (Royal Commission on the National Health Service, 1978b, p.13) agreed with RAWP's view that ameliorating social deprivation was the task of other programmes as a long-term objective (DHSS 1976c, p.11, para. 1.16), but were concerned like clinician critics, about the consequences of reducing health care provision in otherwise deprived areas without any administrative mechanism for ensuring that the deficiencies of the other relevant services would actually be remedied. It was also pointed out that there is no clear distinction between the social and the health functions in society. The remit of the NHS is not so clearly defined. Klein (1977) argued that 'as a matter of fact ... the NHS does at present carry a burden which reflects social conditions rather than their medical consequences.' Thus, there was a contradiction between RAWP's idealism about what should happen and what actually happened at present. By abandoning its social role, the NHS was not going to be able to correct the deficiencies in housing, the environment and employment in deprived areas. Buxton and Klein's criticism of RAWP assumes that social services, etc. are poor in deprived areas which may not be true and ignores the strategic question as to whether health services are an appropriate response to inner city deprivation. Although the NHS may not have had its own administrative device for meeting the problems of the deprived areas, the Working Party would have been aware of the existence at the time of writing its report of a range of inner city social deprivation initiatives taking place in other Government Departments and of the Joint Approach to Social Policy designed to manage the interaction of different welfare programmes. Klein's criticism also overlooked the fact that RAWP was using the SMR specifically as a measure of the relative risk of need between areas. Thus, what was important was the statistical relationship between mortality levels and the prevalence of adverse social conditions.

The debate on the additional pressure imposed on health services in deprived areas rumbled on in the medical press. An editorial in World Medicine (Anonymous, 1978) asked why a composite index of SMRs, morbidity and social deprivation data could not be compiled for use in the formula in the light of Douglas Black's work in developing 'the index of burden' imposed on health services by population disease levels (Black and Pole, 1975). No indication was given of the coherent rationale required to select items for inclusion in such a scale! Avery-Jones (1978 and 1979) reiterated his earlier case based on social conditions in inner London, but extended his argument to stress the supposedly poor quality of general practitioner services in London as a reason for maintaining high levels of funding in hospital services. However no evidence was given of how the primary and secondary care sectors inter-related to impose a greater burden on hospitals in the capital, nor was the problem quantified. It is legitimate to question the brevity and weakness of emphasis in RAWP's discussion of the NHS as an interactive system. The quality of primary and community care may affect the demand for hospital beds and reductions in acute beds could have serious consequences for non-hospital services, especially in deprived inner city areas (Eyles, Smith and Woods, 1982). However, RAWP was limited by its terms of reference to look only at the resources allocated by health authorities. Despite this, the final report does state:

> '..... ways need to be found of securing that the [FPC] resources at present allocated in quite different ways are more closely related so that the impact of geographical disparities in one part of the service or another is taken into account. One way of so doing might be to take account where appropriate of geographic FPS expenditure in determining allocations to Health Authorities. We suggest that a review of the interaction between the two services from a financial viewpoint would be timely ...'
> (DHSS, 1976c, p.81, para. 6.21)

Most recently, local authorities in London have also joined the "social deprivation debate" supporting an allowance for social deprivation as a way of minimising the movement of funds out of inner London and resisting overall NHS cuts (GLC Health Panel, 1984).

A number of observations can be made on these criticisms of RAWP:

1. The sorts of health service and other provision which would actually be relevant to the needs of the socially deprived or which might improve overall community health are never discussed. For example, there is no evidence to suggest that the appropriate response to the excess demand created by poor housing and inadequate GP services is more of what has traditionally been provided, ie. acute hospital beds, as Avery-Jones (1976) conveniently assumed. From her local government perspective, Lally (1980) was almost alone in suggesting that it might be more appropriate to give extra funds to the local authorities in areas where money was being removed through the operation of RAWP, rather than including a social deprivation allowance in Health Service resource allocation.

2. Underlying much of the material is an implicit rejection of a cornerstone of RAWP's thinking on equity; namely, that by far the most important determinant of an area's demand and need for health care is the size and age/sex structure of the population rather than any unique features of its social structure and environment.

3. Much of what appears to be technical criticism conceals a defence of the status quo from those with a direct interest in its maintenance, particularly teaching hospital consultants in London. Such people were disputing the DHSS decision to implement RAWP by holding the over-target RHAs at a standstill in order to provide funds for redistribution on a near static NHS budget (Anonymous, 1976a). Their view was that redistribution should only take place when the national economy allowed "levelling up" on a fast expanding NHS budget. If not, resource inequalities should not be interfered with. Under this approach it is hard to see a time when NHS resources would be sufficiently freely available to allow relatively poorly-off parts of the country to close the gap without any sacrifices by the better off!

4. There is little or no consideration given to the choice of the most appropriate definition of "deprivation" on the basis of existing knowledge about the aetiology of disease. Ideas of "deprivation" developed in other sectors of welfare tend to be borrowed and supported for insertion in the formula, willy-nilly. Much of the debate appears to hinge on how social deprivation is conceptualised. The tendency is for London to be seen as particularly deprived on the basis of unique features of its social structure which may or may not have implications in terms of an increased need for health care.

5. The London centredness of the debate may have been provoked as much by the organisation and quality of primary care services in the capital, as by social and environmental conditions per se. Unfortunately, the areas hypothesised to have poor primary care and socially deprived populations are also the areas with the highest supply of beds and manpower in their respective Regions. Disentangling cause and and effect is therefore difficult when it is known that availability and quality of primary care is likely to affect hospitalisation rates, but so too is the availability and accessibility of hospitals.

6. The debate has been conducted with remarkably little reference to hard evidence concerning the way in which social characteristics of a deprived area influence the need and demand for and use of health services. Little serious thought was given to whether mortality data, as used in RAWP, adequately accounted for deprivation-related differences in health service demand/use. It has also proved extremely difficult to quantify the impact of social deprivation on the NHS, despite calls for attempts to be made (Lally, 1980). In fact, as this Chapter shows, research studies seem generally to agree that mortality and morbidity rates are sufficiently highly associated with a range of indicators of adverse social conditions to be used in resource allocation to Districts.

7. Social indicators are even more indirect proxies for morbidity than mortality rates. They are also only available every ten years, from the Census, whereas mortality data are annual.

RESEARCH ON GEOGRAPHICAL VARIATIONS IN MORTALITY, MORBIDITY AND SOCIAL CONDITIONS

What is the verdict of research since 1976 on complaints about the lack of a social deprivation weighting in RAWP? The RAWP report stimulated interest in an area-based approach to the study of health and social conditions. A number of studies have found statistically significant relationships between various mortality and morbidity indices and a range of selected social indicators, similar to the results of the study used by RAWP. These pieces of research appear to have had little influence on the "RAWP and social deprivation debate". Studies have tended to show that deprived people suffer disadvantage in their health status and make more use of health services than the non-deprived. Yet these features tend to be reflected in their poorer mortality and morbidity, supporting RAWP's decision to use mortality as its principal need weighting after age and sex. The majority of studies show consistent relationships between mortality and morbidity measures and a range of social indicators.

Brennan and Lancashire (1978) found a significant association between early childhood mortality and lower social class, poor housing status (overcrowding, lack of amenities and tenure) and unemployment in County Boroughs in 1971. Forster (1979) looked at the statistical relationships at a Regional level between available health need indices (including both mortality and morbidity data) and 'socio-environmental' indicators. The results did not undermine RAWP's choice of SMRs and in many ways supported RAWP's analysis. For example, the percentage of unskilled manual workers in the population correlated significantly with each of the need measures (mortality rates and acute and chronic sickness from the GHS) as did the percentage unemployed. Similarly, Knox, Marshall, Kane, Green and Mallett (1980) demonstrated strong positive correlations in English AHAs between "expected" perinatal mortality rates (PNMRs) for 1974-6 (calculated by applying national birthweight-specific perinatal mortality rates to local birthweight distributions) and a wide range of variables indicative of poverty and deprivation. Townsend, Simpson and Tibbs (1984) found a strong statistical association between indicators of material deprivation (percentage households with fewer rooms than persons, percentage households lacking a car, percentage unemployed, percentage of children 5-15 years receiving free school meals and percentage of households experiencing disconnection of electricity) and ill-health indicators (stillbirths and infant deaths per 1000 live births, deaths 15-64 years per 1000 of that age, deaths per 1000 65 years and over and low birthweight babies born after 40 weeks' gestation per 1000 births with that gestational period) in Bristol. The two sets of indicators exhibited high rank consistency between wards. The difference for both mortality and low birthweight, between the six least and the six most deprived wards was highly statistically significant.

As a result of their study, Brennan and Lancashire (1978) saw a case for more Health Service investment in areas with higher mortality rates because they also tended to be deprived in Health Service terms as well as socio-economically. Townsend et al (1984) were most modest, concluding that greater efforts should be made to identify and measure the very complex influence of socio-economic conditions on health and the causes of ill-health. However, the implication for RAWP would appear to be that mortality and morbidity indices can adequately take account of deprivation.

Townsend's most recent study of inequalities in health and deprivation in the Northern Region, produces results with similar implications for the "RAWP and social deprivation debate". Using three measures of ill-health (mortality, disablement and delayed development) and four measures of material deprivation (unemployment, non-ownership of a car, non-ownership of a home and overcrowding) combined into two overall indexes at ward level, a highly statistically significant correlation was found between the health index and the deprivation index (Townsend, Phillimore and Beattie, 1986, p.145). Taken alone, mortality, in the form of the O-64 years SMR, was also found to be highly correlated with the deprivation index. Furthermore, in view of the criticism discussed in Chapter Four that SMRs are a poor measure of chronic sickness, SMRs were found to be highly correlated with the disablement measure (percentage of residents permanently sick at the national Census). From these data it would appear that RAWP's choice of the SMR both as a surrogate for morbidity and as a way of encapsulating the effects of deprivation on health, was a sound one, even below District level, contrary to popular mythology in the NHS.

A great variety of structural features of inner city areas and of the health care to be found there, have been viewed as either leading directly to greater morbidity and thence to a greater need for services, or leading indirectly to a greater need for services through the exigencies of poor physical and social conditions. The influential Acheson Report on primary care in London catalogued a long list of social conditions in the inner area which it claimed exerted greater pressure on primary care services, including high population morbidity and the break-up of family networks, the presence of 'vulnerable groups' (alcoholics, ex-mental patients, etc.), one parent families, children in care, poor housing and environment, overcrowding, ethnic minorities, elderly living alone, the proportion of unskilled manual workers, low levels of car ownership, and so on (London Health Planning Consortium, 1981). The Report also pointed to features of health services in inner London which posed particular problems; for instance, the low levels of registration with GPs (due to supposed difficulties of access to the limited lists of part-time GPs) were associated with a higher than average demand on accident and emergency services; the poor quality of community support services for the elderly and of GP care were related by the authors to extra pressure on hospital care. The Report cited possible problems encountered by primary care personnel in inner London, namely the risk of attack, vandalism to premises and equipment and difficulties in gaining access to patients because of traffic congestion. However, little of the material put forward to Acheson could be said to have been based on rigorous research. It is impossible to tell precisely what impact the inner city factors quoted by Acheson were likely to have on the need for hospital resorces.

Detailed local studies are required to substantiate the case put in the Acheson report. In one of the very few studies based on a community morbidity survey, Skrimshire (1978) compared morbidity in three contrasting, but socially homogeneous small areas with high, average and low SMRs respectively: a new working class council estate in socially deprived Newham, London; a "problem" working class council estate in a then prosperous part of the Midlands; and a prosperous middle class owner-occupied district in the same part of the Midlands. Although the self-reported morbidity of the three areas tended to mirror their local mortality rates, thus supporting RAWP's use of mortality data as an overall need proxy, there was some evidence of a possible environmental effect increasing child morbidity in the socially deprived area which was not picked up in mortality rates. The inference seemed to be that it might be necessary to consider inclusion in RAWP of social and especially environmental factors over and above mortality, at least for children. Using a different methodology Brennan and Lancashire (1978) found a similar 'area effect' for child mortality under five years. A highly significant association remained between child mortality and housing density and facilities when social class and unemployment were controlled for.

Skrimshire (1978) also looked at use of and quality of interaction with, primary care in the three neighbourhoods and found a contrast between the two working class samples and the middle class sample. Reported difficulties and distress in communication with GPs and other health workers and in the way the general practices managed appointments, emergencies, etc. and lower overall satisfaction with primary care were more common in the working class patients. There was some evidence that the level of primary care manpower in relation to the workload was lower in the working class areas. Skrimshire also makes the important suggestion that not only does social class disadvantage affect levels of health behaviour and demand among patients, but it may also interact with and exacerbate problems in the relationships between individuals and their GPs. Specifically, Skrimshire suggests that working class patients lack the skills to communicate problems effectively to the doctor and that the greater 'social distance' between GPs and working class patients in terms of their differing values, assumptions and experiences works against a satisfactory relationship as perceived by the working class patient. In summary, Skrimshire's 'area hypothesis' is:

'... that health, the provision of health care and the subjective experience of seeking that care are all partly determined by the socio-economic structure of society on an area basis, so that a working class person is at a greater disadvantage if he lives in a predominantly working class area than if he lives in a socially mixed area. The data ... are consistent with a theory of structural determination of need and demand for health care from an area, operating both through environmental and social conditions on the level of health and through the social pressures and life experiences that further affect demand, particularly in cases of childhood illness. The level and quality of available medical manpower, relative to need and demand, is likely also to be strongly affected by the environment and social class composition of an area through the operation of the market for recruitment.'
(Skrimshire, 1978, p.51)

The policy implications which Skrimshire draws from her analysis are:

1. If the 'area hypothesis' holds, there is justification for a policy of positive discrimination of primary care resources in favour of socially and environmentally deprived areas to counteract some of the conditions under which doctors operate in deprived areas and the market forces which affect recruitment.

2. However, health services resource allocation policies are of limited scope and effect against the structural determination of levels of health and patterns of health service use in deprived areas. Policies to modify poverty, poor housing and environmental hazards may be more appropriate.

3. Need indicators for use in resource allocation should relate clearly to areas of a size at which relevant environmental and structural factors are likely to operate (ie. possibly at sub-District level).

On balance, Skrimshire's studies illuminate the particular needs for health care in small areas, but not surprisingly for a pilot study yield few firm guides to the debate on whether and how social deprivation should be taken into account in calculating the need for health service resources at the level of District Health Authorities. The most interesting result in Skrimshire's study from a RAWP perspective was the finding that the self-reported morbidity levels in the three small areas corresponded with their relative mortality positions, implying that mortality data were a reasonable proxy for morbidity and social conditions.

The relationship between area deprivation, use of services and health is complex. Data on access to and quality of primary care require careful interpretation. Thus Knox showed that access to primary care was high in the inner city areas of Scottish cities (which were among the most deprived neighbourhoods) and low in the peripheral zones of public housing (also deprived), but that the inner city areas seemed to be worst-off in terms of the quality of primary care services (Knox, 1978; Knox, 1979).

A number of other studies have focused more directly on quantifying the relationship between socio-economic factors, morbidity and use of health services. For example, Scott-Samuel (1977) examined variation in health data for clusters of small areas in Liverpool, using a socio-economic typology developed by OPCS ('social area analysis'). Infant mortality, uptake of vaccination and incidence of infectious disease were higher in clusters with a higher proportion in social classes IV and V. The implication was that social area analysis based on suitable variables could be undertaken to establish resource or service needs for different types of area in place of using SMRs. However, the clusters of 'social areas' used were not ranged by degree of deprivation as much as by differences in social, housing and other features Thus, it is difficult to argue that the results indicate the need for a social deprivation weight in RAWP.

An area-based study employing a composite index of deprivation was carried out by Carstairs (1981). She examined whether populations in deprived areas had higher morbidity by correlating a composite deprivation index (derived by correlating individual deprivation variables and health indicators) with a range of health indicators (deaths, discharges and bed days) for wards in Glasgow and Edinburgh. For much of the data, including mortality and deprivation (as assumed by RAWP), the associations were fairly strong, as expected, and indicated greater "need" in areas of greater deprivation. The question remained however, as to the contribution of factors other than morbidity to service use and need; namely, the level of bed provision, quality of primary care and other social factors not necessarily reflected in morbidity and therefore, the need to take account of these in RAWP. Bed provision and quality of primary care did not appear to be important in this case but there was some evidence of the operation of social factors over and above morbidity in deprived areas. For example, length of stay in hospital was longer in the more deprived categories, although this could have been due to differences in the severity of cases between more and less deprived areas. Thus, true differences in morbidity could still be the explanation, for which mortality data are a reasonable proxy, as was seen in Chapter Four.

Although the correlation of the health indicator of deaths (0-64 years) was very slightly higher with the composite deprivation index than with any of the individual deprivation variables, it did not appear that the composite measure had much to offer over the individual deprivation variables in explanatory power in relation to the health indicators. Since the social class variable (percentage of the population in social class V) correlated very highly with most of the other individual deprivation variables, Carstairs (1981) was forced to conclude that the concept of deprivation may have little to add to the well known associations between morbidity and social class. However, her analysis was not capable of conclusively answering the question of whether there is an 'area effect' attributable to deprivation, over and above that predicted by the social class composition of the population.

A similar analysis for local authority areas in North Western RHA by Johnson used three variables and a clustering technique to group areas into six classes which exhibited a considerable gradient in deprivation. SMRs and bed use increased throughout the deprivation gradient (Carstairs, 1982). The marked association between mortality and deprivation in this analysis would tend to support RAWP's decision to use mortality data. It would appear that deprivation is ultimately reflected in the morbidity and mortality levels in a population. However, the results of this type of analysis have had scarcely any influence on the debate within the NHS on RAWP and social deprivation, which has been sustained by the complaints of the RAWP-losing Districts.

THE APPLICATION OF SOCIAL INDICATORS IN SUB-REGIONAL RAWP

The absence of a social deprivation weight from sub-Regional RAWP was taken up not only by clinicians, but also by officials in inner city Districts which stood to gain by the inclusion of such an allowance. In response to NHS political pressure, a number of Regions in London have amended their sub-Regional RAWP formulae accordingly (National Association of Health Authorities, 1983). The rationale appeared to be that the "health deprived" were concentrated geographically in particular Districts and that additional funding could improve their health care and ultimately, their health status. This was similar to the spatial policies of positive discrimination devised in the 1960s in other areas of social policy (eg. education and housing). These policies had been increasingly discredited as inefficient in targeting resources on the needy and based in doubtful theories of deprivation by the time they were taken up in the Health Service!

A number of different replacements for SMRs have been proposed and will be reviewed.

The DHSS/Thames Regions' Joint Working Group

The initial response of the Thames Regions to deprivation was crude. In 1978, North East Thames RHA increased its acute hospital bed norm from 2.5 beds per 1000 population to 3.0 per 1000 for the inner city AHAs. It was recognised that this move was not justified by a proper analysis. Accordingly, a Joint Working Group of DHSS together with the four Thames Regions, was convened to consider, among other matters, whether it would be possible and justifiable to devise a more sophisticated deprivation adjustment to the RAWP formula for the Thames Regions (DHSS and Thames Regional Health Authorities, 1979). The Working Group began by examining the relationship between condition-aggregated SMRs and various social deprivation indicators to determine if SMRs adequately mirrored deprivation. Three indicators were chosen (percentage of New Commonwealth immigrants, percentage of households lacking exclusive use of a basic amenity and percentage of pensioners living alone) on the basis of the impact they might be expected to make on need for health services. There was some correlation with SMRs, but there was sufficient discrepancy for the Working Group to conclude that deprivation should be accounted for independently of SMRs. Thus, a simple classification of AHAs into "high", "medium" or "low" deprivation according to how they scored on the three deprivation variables was devised. The Working Group recommended using the score to weight the populations used to calculate the NPIP, day and outpatient, ambulance and community health services' targets. The effect of the suggested weightings was to increase the targets of the "high" deprivation AHAs by 5%, the "medium" AHAs by 3% and the "low" AHAs remained unchanged. The weightings were apparently cross-checked against known health service utilisation rates to the satisfaction of the Working Group. The validity of the classification was also tested by matching the three groups of boroughs against a cluster analysis of 23 social indicators undertaken by Valerie Imber to compile A Classification of English Personal Social Services Authorities which grouped authorities in terms of their social conditions associated with demand for social services (DHSS, 1977b). The cluster analysis matched the three groups very closely. The Joint Working Group (JWG) did not have time or the necessary data to consider issues such as the possible existence of sub-District pockets of severe deprivation or the effect of supply factors such as the availability of GP services on the need for hospital and community health services.

On the basis of the above analysis some of the Thames Regions adopted a social deprivation weighting in their sub-Regional RAWP formula in addition to SMRs.

Yet the methods and assumptions used in the DHSS/Thames Regions' report were extremely unsophisticated. One commentator sums up his criticism as follows:

'... the method ... is not only distinguished by the arbitrary selection of deprivation indicators and population weightings, but by the adoption of a policy of areally based positive discrimination which ignores recent research on the efficiency of such policies to meet the needs of the majority of the socially deprived. Further, whilst the Working Group is prepared to discriminate in favour of certain area health authorities it does not consider the issue of how additional resources could be used to meet the needs of the socially deprived in those authorities.' (Woods, 1982, p.79)

There were a large number of problems with the DHSS/Thames Regions' approach. They will be discussed in some detail since similar drawbacks occur in more sophisticated, later analyses:

1. The three social deprivation indicators were chosen arbitrarily on the basis of their likely impact on need for health care and to be representative of other social deprivation indicators. However, no indication is given in the report as to why the three were chosen in preference to others, nor how their association with health need was established (DHSS and Thames Regional Health Authorities, 1979). There are no references in the report to any of the studies available at that time which had attempted to look at the relationship between morbidity and social factors (eg. Brennan and Lancashire, 1978).

There appears to have been no analysis of the likely inter-correlation of the three variables and no discussion of whether they did indeed measure social deprivation, since the Working Group did not appear to regard it as necessary to define the concept of "social deprivation" which it was using. It would seem reasonable that different concepts should be used in health planning than say education or housing. Social deprivation was defined pragmatically as the presence of the three selected variables. Yet it is doubtful if any of the three can accurately be described as a "deprivation variable" at all (see the concluding section of this Chapter for a further discussion of this).

2. Even if the three variables adequately defined social deprivation, the variables had to be weighted for use in RAWP. The report does not make it clear how the weightings were arrived at except that they were cross-checked against known utilisation rates. The fact that the two sets of data corresponded was taken to be an indication that it was appropriate to use the three variables selected. One must presume that this was because the weightings matched the subjective judgement of the Group as to which AHAs were more or less "socially deprived" (Woods, 1982). Yet utilisation data are inappropriate to validate a measure of need.

3. The Joint Working Group implicitly assumed that the socially deprived were concentrated in inner London. Woods (1982) quotes research from the mid-1970s showing that on the contrary, the spatial concentration of deprivation was quite low and cites, as an example, the basic flaw in the Education Priority Areas (EPAs) strategy (another area-based attempt at positive discrimination through resource allocation) in which it was found that the majority of the individuals whom the scheme was aimed at, lived outside the designated EPAs. Proportional data can mislead by giving the impression that a group within a defined area is larger than it is, particularly when the population denominator is small. Analysis of the spatial distribution of the populations associated with the three variables chosen by the JWG in the four Thames Regions showed that in no case did the proportion of households in the so called "high" deprivation areas exhibiting the three deprivation characteristics (households headed by someone from the New Commonwealth, households lacking use of a basic amenity and lone

pensioner households) exceed 45% of the total of such households. In fact, more lone pensioners lived in the "low" deprivation areas than in the "high" deprivation areas (Woods, 1982). These results reflected the fact that more people lived outside than inside the "deprived" areas.

4. The JWG chose to assume that socially deprived areas need more health services. It also adopted RAWP's assumption that spending more on areas lacking in health services would ensure that they received more and better services. The allowance for deprivation which resulted from the JWG's recommendations was to be part of the general allocation of revenue to health authorities and was not earmarked for particular schemes. The JWG did not question whether the prevailing balance and structure of inner city health services were appropriate for the needs of the local population and made no recommendations as to how services should be changed in return for receiving extra money for social deprivation. It was as if the JWG accepted the status quo argument that more hospital beds could form an interim solution to the problem of the demands placed on the NHS by inner city deprivation, until, in the long-term, the social environment could be improved (Avery-Jones, 1976).

5. A major weakness of the JWG's analysis (and of more sophisticated ones in the same vein) is the absence of any means of taking account of the interaction of deprivation and health service supply variables which may confound any relationship established betweeen deprivation and need for health services. It is known from research in the 1960s that in localities with more hospital beds, hospitalisation rates are higher than in places with fewer beds, regardless of social conditions (Feldstein, 1965; Feldstein, 1967) and that cases tend to be admitted for longer periods of time (Logan, Ashley, Klein and Robson, 1972). The inner London AHAs which exhibit features of social deprivation also happen to have more health service resources (especially beds) than other parts of England because of the number of large teaching hospitals. Thus, it is essential to be able to make some estimate of the relative contribution of high levels of supply and social deprivation to the historic pattern of utilisation, before recommending amendments to the RAWP formula. Otherwise there is a risk that a spurious relationship will be used to justify a dilution of the process of equitable redistribution.

6. The JWG presented its recommendations disingenuously as if they were the result of a purely technical exercise. The report exudes pseudo-objectivity, but makes no mention of the political pressures surrounding resource allocation in the Thames Regions which inevitably influenced analysis of the issues. Perhaps because of this, the report's recommendations were very successful both politically and administratively: they went some way to answering the inner London critics of RAWP who regarded the formula as insensitive to their particular needs, by giving them extra funds; and they satisfied the remaining AHAs by their "rational", "objective" methodology.

The Black Report and RAWP

In contrast to the pragmatic over-simplification of the DHSS/Thames Regions JWG, the Black Report on inequalities in health addressed the same question of whether there were 'area indicators of social deprivation which might be used independently or in supplementation of SMRs in developing a [sub-Regional] formula for resource allocation' (DHSS, 1980a, p.254). The Black Report looked in a more sophisticated way than the JWG at the Census variables relevant to need for social services (and by extension, therefore, health services) used by Imber (DHSS, 1977b). 'Overcrowding' had the highest correlation with the other deprivation variables, rather than any of the three chosen by the JWG. The Black Report also took full account unlike the JWG, of a range of epidemiological studies on the association between social variables and mortality rates. For example, Black and colleagues were aware that Brennan and

Lancashire (1978) had shown that areas with high unemployment or bad housing or a high proportion of the population in social class V (or worst, all three) were highly likely to have high rates of child mortality. The Black Research Working Group agreed that such data would tend to support the case for using a single mortality indicator (such as the SMR) in resource allocation, since mortality and social conditions co-varied in a number of studies. However, the Working Party did not find the evidence conclusive in this direction, but preferred 'to keep an open mind' (DHSS, 1980a, p.261) until more work had been undertaken to develop social indicators which specifically reflected health service needs. Although social factors were reflected in high mortality rates, it was also possible that they might increase the need for care among survivors. On the other hand, this suggestion was not proven either! Nevertheless, the Black Research Working Group was prepared to concede the possibility that a combination of SMRs and other social measures might produce, 'more satisfactory, and administratively and politically defensible results' (DHSS, 1980a, p.261) and went on:

> 'Our argument is that by also taking account of population and community characteristics (other than age/sex) indicative of need for care, as well as physical amenities and evironmental conditions, a better overall measure of need for resources can be produced. This is not easy to prove since there is no direct measure of need which would permit regression of SMR (and any alternative measure of morbidity or health) and social conditions together.' (DHSS, 1980a, p.261)

The Black Report's contribution is significant because it recognises the political and value-laden nature of the argument over social deprivation in RAWP and the great difficulty of proving one approach a fairer depiction of reality than another, since we lack a direct measure of need. Whichever weighting is chosen, by definition, a formula is somewhat arbitrary. However, the Black Research Working Group maintained that weightings should, as far as possible, be derived from available empirical material, in contrast to the a priori reasoning of the four Thames Regions and DHSS. For example, the community health services component of the RAWP formula allowed for population age/sex structure and SMR only, but Brennan and Lancashire (1978) had shown that in areas of overcrowding, high unemployment, or with a high percentage of the population in social class V, children aged 0-4 years ran particular health risks. Based on this sort of evidence, the Black Research Working Group recommended that the population 0-4 years should be weighted according to the levels of overcrowding , unemployment or numbers of unskilled manual workers in the population (taking account of inter-correlations) for the purposes of calculating the element of the RAWP target for community health services.

The Black Report left researchers with the challenge of pursuing more sustained and subtle comparisons of different measures of social or occupational class and health need and particularly the development of social indicators which genuinely related to a theory of health service needs (DHSS, 1980a, p.261). However, subsequent analysis in the NHS has shown that this is a formidable task which depends as much on an adequate theoretical perspective as on complex data manipulation. For example, recent work by Dearden using conventional data sources and standard correlational methods in which Regional level data from the GHS on selected health variables are "fitted" onto a range of 1981 Census social variables, appears to offer little improvement on the numerous studies reported above (Dearden, 1985, pp.11-12). If there is a reasonable "fit" with certain social variables, Dearden proposes using these variables in RAWP target simulations along with tests of the effect of alternative mortality indices. There is no sign that Dearden is doing more than performing a correlation analysis on existing variables and calling this "deprivation". This is despite the fact that he quotes with approval Edwards' recommendation of ten years ago concerning social indicators and deprivation. Edwards argued that we should start with our own specific concept of deprivation, appropriate to the particular service or source of deprivation, rather than arriving at a notion of deprivation based on a correlation study of available social indicators (Edwards, 1975). While Edwards' approach tends towards arbitrariness unless prefaced by a thorough review of the available evidence, Dearden's verges on serendipity.

The North Thames Regions' Inpatient Census: Socio-Economic Group Weightings

An alternative approach which moves the debate forward, but does not require an elaborate concept of health deprivation is the census of health service utilisation. Officials in the Thames Regions were well aware of the limitations of the methods used by the DHSS/Thames RHAs Joint Working Group in 1979 to identify three arbitrary social deprivation variables for inclusion in RAWP (DHSS and Thames Regional Health Authorities, 1979). They wished for a better way to identify a more appropriate proxy for morbidity than SMRs for use in RAWP, but one which was also independent of supply. The long-term solution to providing acceptable morbidity measures was seen to lie with frequent morbidity surveys of needs relevant to NHS provision, based on large samples of health authority populations. However, this was not feasible through lack of resources. A hospital inpatient census was fixed on by North West and North East Thames RHAs as an interim solution to the problem of bridging the gap between data on utilisation and data on socio-economic conditions for resource allocation purposes. There was limited evidence in the Thames Regions of increased hospital utilisation rates in areas of social deprivation and pressure from AHAs with potentially high deprivation scores for greater recognition of this in sub-Regional RAWP. The problem for the RHAs was the association between areas of social deprivation and areas with a high level of supply of hospital resources. Hence the attraction of a bed census since it would yield data directly relevant to utilisation, while at the same time some allowance could conceivably be made for the relevant effects of social deprivation and the supply of hospital beds. The aim would be to describe the relative utilisation of inpatient services by groups with known social characteristics and availability of supply.

In the inpatient census which was carried out in Autumn 1981 in the two North Thames Regions all patients in non-psychiatric, acute beds (excluding maternity beds) on a specified day, were surveyed using questions about personal and social circumstances from the 1981 national Census and including additional questions about dependency and reason for admission. These data were linked to Hospital Activity Analysis (HAA) and national Census data for the relevant Districts. Age/sex standardised hospital utilisation rates were computed for persons with a range of social characteristics (New Commonwealth immigrant, social class, socio-economic group, employment status, lack of exclusive use of basic amenities and elderly living alone) and the social characteristics of the inpatient population compared with the total population from which they were drawn.

The principal findings in the NE and NW Thames censuses were as follows (North East Thames Regional Health Authority, 1983a and 1983b; North West Thames Regional Health Authority, undated):

1. For patients under 65, there was little appreciable difference in length of stay between New Commonwealth-born and UK born patients (there were too few elderly New Commonwealth patients to make comparisons).

2. Age/sex standardised admission rates correlated significantly with the two occupational classifications of social class (0.65) and socio-economic group (SEG) (0.63) at DHA level. At local authority level, the best correlation was with SEG (0.69) followed by social class (0.64). SEG was to be preferred to social class because it included the retired who are heavy users of the NHS.

3. Correlations of bed use with 'lack of basic amenities' were statistically significant, but since SEG and lack of basic amenities were highly inter-correlated, this implied that they were measuring similar population characteristics. As a resource allocation variable, 'lack of basic amenities' had the disadvantage of referring to only a small proportion of the population.

4. The variable 'elderly living alone' only had significant impact on bed utilisation in the three inner London Districts. It was difficult to assess the extent to which this reflected the effect of inner city multiple deprivation and might therefore be accounted for by the SEG structure of the population.

It was concluded that SEG was the most powerful explanatory social variable in accounting statistically for variation in hospital bed utilisation next to the age/sex structure of the population. In an attempt to correct for differences in the supply characteristics of each District, NE Thames analysts looked at the gradient in the relationship between SEG composition of the population and the standardised bed utilisation rate between inner London, outer London and the county Districts within the Region. The observed consistency of the gradient between the three groups of Districts was offered as evidence that the SEG factor was independent of supply and could therefore be used in RAWP as a proxy for morbidity. Interestingly, the SEG composition of a District was also found to be independent of the District SMR values which would have been used in conventional RAWP.

The SEG weightings derived from the relative hospital utilisation of different SEG categories, varied by 17% at the extremes between Districts in NE Thames RHA. Thus SEG structure discriminated much more sharply between inner city, suburban and Home Counties' Districts than the social deprivation weightings produced by the three social deprivation variables used in the 1979 Thames Regional analysis which varied by only 5% (DHSS and Thames Regional Health Authorities, 1979).

The 1981 North Thames inpatient censuses represent an important body of research generated within the NHS which has been inadequately written up and publicised both to academics and practitioners. It represents an attempt to disentangle supply (beds) factors from demand (social) factors in determining hospital utilisation rates, using data rigorously collected from a large number of cases. However, the North Thames censuses are only a starting point, since they are based on utilisation data. Ultimately, the measure of morbidity used in the censuses depends on the existence of beds to which patients can be admitted. Remove the beds and the morbidity cannot be recorded! Direct comparisons between population-based data on morbidity and the incidence and prevalence of a range of conditions and the use of facilities by the same populations, would be required to reach more definitive conclusions about the effect of supply on the relationship between social conditions, demand and need for health services.

Following the two North Thames patient censuses, both the North Thames RHAs have chosen to use a utilisation-weighted index of District SEG composition as the combined morbidity and social conditions weighting in their sub-Regional RAWP formulae (NPIP, outpatient/day patient, ambulance and community services elements) in place of SMRs. This also supercedes the previous social deprivation weights determined by the DHSS/Thames Regions Joint Working Group in 1979. For example, in North East Thames RHA, the percentage deprivation weights of the inner London DHAs (Region = 0%) are, Tower Hamlets, 10.5%, Newham, 7.6%, City and Hackney 6.8% and Islington 6.6%. The SEG weighting was first implemented in North East Thames RHA in 1984/85. Without carrying out its own census, South West Thames RHA has also taken up the results of the North Thames censuses and now includes SEGs in its RAWP formula. The SEG utilisation weightings have been derived from North West Thames data because it was felt that the two populations corresponded more closely than would have been the case with North East Thames data. The Region has also looked at the possibility of including the number of elderly living alone as an additional weighting since in the North West Thames census 'elderly living alone' appeared to contribute independently to bed utilisation in the inner London DHAs. South West Thames took GHS data on the prevalence of elderly people living alone with 'long standing illness, disability or infirmity' and prepared weightings which were applied to the estimated numbers of elderly living alone in DHAs in 1993. The impact on Districts' targets was very slight (Dowie, 1985).

The inclusion of SEGs in sub-Regional RAWP in three of the Thames RHAs has had the effect of increasing the targets for the over-target Districts which tend to have a higher proportion of their populations in the lower SEGs, while decreasing the targets of under-target DHAs. This reduces the amount of revenue which needs to be redistributed between Districts within these Regions to achieve RAWP-defined equity and protects a greater proportion of the revenue of the teaching Districts than previously. This is likely to have contributed to the attractiveness of the policy of including SEGs. It has enabled three Thames Regions to respond to political pressure from the influential inner London Districts to reduce the scale of redistribution on grounds of social conditions, while satisfying other Districts by maintaining an overall policy of equitable redistribution. It is interesting to note that a social deprivation weighting has only been included in sub-Regional RAWP in the Thames Regions, despite the existence of deprived inner city areas in all Regions (National Association of Health Authorities, 1983).

The principal weakness of the North Thames methodology lies in the difficulty of controlling for supply. Recent research by Cullis, Forster and Frost (1981) demonstrates the importance of supply effects. Cullis et al investigated the relationship between SMRs, bed supply, admission rates and bed use rates between the English RHAs and also within Trent RHA. They found that the largest percentage of the observed variation in admission rates could be explained in terms of bed supply, confirming earlier work by Logan et al (1972). The relationships of admission rates to SMRs were insignificant and weaker after controlling for available beds, particularly sub-Regionally. SMR did not appear strongly to influence the demand for hospital care. There is no reason to expect that it would. These results are a reminder that data on use of services are always going to be difficult to interpret as proxies for "need". In other recent work, Carstairs (1981) in Glasgow found that the inter-related variables of unemployment and proportion of the population in Social Class V had a higher correlation with bed days than an overall index of social deprivation, lending some support to the North Thames Regions' decision to use an index of class structure rather than social deprivation in RAWP. On the other hand, Fox and Golblatt (1982) and Morgan (1983) adduce evidence which would suggest that housing tenure and car ownership are more closely associated with mortality and morbidity rates than occupationally-based measures of social class or socio-economic group. However, the North Thames Censuses showed otherwise for use of hospital services. It is unsurprising that the findings of these studies are not consistent, since they employ a variety of different proxies for health need. There is no reason to expect that a measure of demand (adjusted for the availability of health resources) used as a proxy for need, should bear the same relationship to social conditions as measures of morbidity or mortality, used as need proxies.

Weightings Based on an Area Classification of Residential Neighbourhoods (ACORN)

Since 1981, there has been interest in alternatives to conventional ways of studying social inequality and its relationship with health need and health service use. Health service planners have become interested in the concept of targeting services on groups which may be particularly at risk, but have lacked the detailed spatial tools to be able to identify groups with different social characteristics and different patterns of health and health service use. It has been argued that traditional, single indicator, occupational, classifications do not provide specific information on the features of people's lifestyle, resources and environment which are likely to be implicated in their need for health services. Furthermore, they are problematic when applied to women, single parent families, retired people and the unemployed. Morgan (1983) reviewed a range of different measures of social inequality (single indicator and composite measures, including area-based measures) which are capable of identifying groups which differ in their health experience and health service use (and therefore, need). The main disadvantage of occupational classifications lay in obtaining sufficiently precise information for classification and in the increasing complexity of coding occupational data as the employment structure of society becomes more and more highly differentiated. Educational attainment classifications were important in distinguishing between different attitudes and behavioural patterns of individuals, while housing tenure classifications tended to emphasise economic resources. Area-based classifications had the potential to identify groups which were particularly deprived in health terms since they combined socio-economic characteristics of individuals with features of their environment. (It had been indicated in a number of studies that a social deprivation effect on sickness operated over and above better-known social class effects (eg. Skrimshire, 1978)). Morgan distinguished purposive classifications such as Carstairs' nine deprivation categories (Carstairs, 1981) which are intended to rank groups along a particular dimension such as social deprivation, from pragmatic classifications such as Scott-Samuels' analysis of family types (Scott-Samuel, 1977) and ACORN 'A Classification of Residential Neighbourhoods', which are descriptive and identify unranked groups comprising areas regarded as homogeneous in their socio-economic conditions.

ACORN was originally devised as a commercial marketing and market research instrument to identify small residential neighbourhoods with homogeneous, but distinctive lifestyle and consumer habits. It consists of eleven unranked ACORN groups* (or in more detail, 36 ACORN Types) comprising distinct types of neighbourhoods derived from a cluster analysis of 40 variables from the 1981 Census relating to six sorts of social indices (age structure, employment, family structure, type of housing, social status and car ownership). Each Enumeration District in the country can thus be assigned to an ACORN Group and ACORN Type according to its Census social characteristics and any individual can be assigned to an ACORN Group or ACORN Type from his/her postcode.

Tests have been made of ACORN's ability to discriminate between the health experience of different groups in the population. Morgan and Chinn (1983)

---

* The ACORN Groups are as follows: A Agricultural; B Modern family housing, higher incomes; C older housing of intermediate status; D Poor quality older terraced housing; E Better-off council estates; F less well-off council estates; G Poorest council estates; H multi-racial areas; I High status non-family areas; J Affluent suburban housing; K Better-off retirement areas.

compared ACORN with the Registrar General's social class classification using health data from a national sample of 5,500 primary school children. Eleven ACORN Groups differentiated at least as well as social class on seven selected outcome measures, identifying the poorest health experience or the highest service use in each case. By using 36 ACORN Types (from which the 11 Acorn Groups are built) and postcodes of children, small areas whose children were extremely disadvantaged in terms of health outcomes were able to be located. This ability to distinguish health-disadvantaged areas makes ACORN a potentially helpful tool for planning, resource allocation and service delivery. It has the practical advantages that it applies to all groups in the population unlike a number of other social deprivation measures, requires only a postcode for classification of an individual and uses the Enumeration District as its building block, enabling a very detailed picture of an area to be compiled. However, the analysis by Morgan and Chinn (1983) raised the question of whether the differentiation achieved by ACORN reflected predominantly regional differences which were to some degree independent of social class, since the distribution of ACORN groups varies markedly by region. Subsequent research examined whether ACORN differentiated on selected mortality indicators within South West Thames RHA. ACORN Groups identified a considerable range in SMRs, suggesting that ACORN Groups identified populations which differed in their health experience even within a single Region. The mortality rates for conditions which generally exhibit a negative social class gradient (eg. bronchitis and heart disease) were highest in ACORN Group G (the poorest council estates) which covered localities with the poorest socio-economic conditions in the Region. (Social Medicine and Health Services Research Unit, 1985, pp. 60-63). This analysis therefore suggests that the variation explained by ACORN and its ability to identify high risk groups is unlikely to be due to the effect of geographical clustering of ACORN Groups and that ACORN identifies consistent variations in health, independent of regional variations. This was further confirmed by an analysis of the distribution of ACORN Groups among the DHAs of South East Thames RHA which showed there to be a considerable spread of most, but not all, ACORN Groups in each District, including Group G (the poorest council estates) with the poorest socio-economic conditions. The spread of ACORN Groups is important for its general use as an indicator of health need in the NHS.

There is an obvious application of ACORN in health promotion campaigns and in targeting services at a local level to meet the needs of groups with high morbidity and low service uptake and possibly also in aetiological studies of specific diseases associated with distinct types of neighbourhoods (Speller and Hale, 1985). However, for this discussion, the main application is as a potential weighting for social conditions in sub-Regional RAWP, since it is repeatedly argued, particularly by inner city DHAs, that the economic and social circumstances of their patients both increase their clinical need for services and place greater demands on health services in meeting such need than would be the case elsewhere. ACORN is attractive because it offers a wide ranging indicator of socio-economic conditions and requires only postcode data from patients. However, it has to be remembered that ACORN is a classification of the characteristics of areas which are distinct from the characteristics of the individuals living in those areas. Knowledge of the area in which someone lives does not necessarily make it possible to predict their health experience. If possible, it is preferable to have data on the circumstances of individuals (eg. their housing tenure) to measure their risk of needing health care rather than to have to rely on surrogates (Fox, Jones and Goldblatt, 1984).

Nevertheless, South East Thames RHA has begun development work on the use of ACORN for its sub-Regional RAWP procedure. Patients using hospital inpatient, community nursing, maternity, outpatient and accident and emergency services

across South East Thames were surveyed in order to study differences in demand
(utilisation) by ACORN Group. The results indicate that ACORN Group appears to
identify differences in the demand for health care between geographical areas
and may, therefore, be useful in sub-Regional resource allocation (South East
Thames Regional Health Authority, 1985). However, a number of DHAs had to be
excluded from the analysis because of high outflows to other Regions for which
ACORN data were not available.

The inpatient deaths and discharges (D & D) rate was highest for Group G
(poorest council estates), followed by H (multi-racial areas) and F (less
well-off council estates). The lowest inpatient D & D rate was in A
(agricultural areas). There appeared to be a relationship (as one would expect)
between the level of provision in a District as measured by available beds per
1000 resident population and the D & D rate of ACORN Groups in that District:
the "high provision" Districts exhibited the highest D & D rates within each
ACORN Group with the exception of A (agricultural). The relative contribution
to D & D rate of age, sex, provision and ACORN Group was modelled
mathematically. Predictably, the age structure of the population was the most
important factor determining the D & D rate, but levels of provision and ACORN
Group also appeared to affect the D & D rate appreciably. The surveys of
maternity and community nursing services revealed similar consistently high or
low use of health services between ACORN Groups.

In view of these results, a methodology has been developed for devising ACORN
weights with the recommendation that ACORN should be incorporated in
sub-Regional RAWP within South East Thames RHA in place of SMRs and SFRs
(standardised fertility ratios for use in the maternity services' element of the
target) (South East Thames Regional Health Authority, 1986a).

The most fundamental problem in deriving weightings from ACORN Group age-and-sex
specific utilisation rates is the familiar and intractable one of making
sensible allowances for the effect on utilisation of variations in the existing
level of service provision in Districts. For example, the D & D rate for ACORN
Group A (agricultural areas) was the lowest of the 11 Groups. It is very likely
that this reflects the fact that the vast majority of Enumeration Districts
within Acorn Group A are in country areas relatively remote from centres of
population and therefore, with poorer access to hospitals. When the D & D rate
for ACORN Group A is sub-divided into "high", "medium" and "low" provision
Districts on the basis of a crude bed availability factor, it is interesting to
note that A is the only ACORN Group in which the "high" provision Districts' D &
D rate is lower than the D & D rates for the "medium" provision Districts. In
all the other Acorn Groups the D & D rate in the "high" provision Districts is
much higher than in either the "medium" or "low" provision Districts. One
possible explanation for this is the likely small number of cases from
agricultural EDs in "high" provision Districts. It is possible that this
analysis by SE Thames RHA exaggerates the homogeneity of Districts with respect
to ACORN Group, since it omits among others, two inner city DHAs, West Lambeth
and Camberwell, which are likely to be untypical of the majority of Districts in
the Region. Some ACORN Groups may be completely absent from particular
Districts (eg. ACORN Group H, multi-racial areas, is probably heavily
concentrated in the inner cities).

South East Thames RHA looked at the effect of supply on utilisation by comparing
D & D rates by ACORN Group between "high", "medium" and "low" provision
Districts (South East Thames RHA, 1985). Bed supply had a marked impact on D &
D rates since the "high" provision Districts showed higher D & D rates than
"medium" or "low" provision Districts for all but one of the ACORN Groups.
However, when considering the effect of supply in the "medium" and "low"
provision Districts it was apparent that the impact of supply varied depending
on ACORN Group. For instance, in Groups D (poor quality older terraced

housing), G (poorest council estates), I (high status non-family areas) and K (better-off retirement areas), the "low" provision Districts had higher D & D rates than the "medium" provision Districts. This is particularly the case for G and I. Unfortunately, this may be an artefact of the analysis since the D & D rates used take no account of the age/sex structure of the ACORN Group population and thus the analysis is inadequate even as a starting point for speculation about supply effects (South East Thames Regional Health Authority, 1985). As a minimum what is required is to study the consistency of the relationships between the age/sex standardised D & D rates for each of the eleven ACORN Groups across the three provision bands of "high", "medium" and "low". From this it should be possible to see whether in relative terms, ACORN Group exerts the same influence on D & D rates in widely different circumstances of bed availability. However, this still does not solve the problem that each Group may be unequally distributed across Districts with different supply characteristics. The South East Thames proposals for devising ACORN weights for use in RAWP compensate for supply by taking the usage rate for each ACORN group to be the midpoint between the rates in "high" and "low" provision Districts (South East Thames Regional Health Authority, 1986a). However, this does not satisfactorily overcome this limitation in the application of ACORN. The same problem occurs in all analyses which rely on use of services data as a basis for an alternative to SMRs. Indeed, even if the distribution of ACORN Groups (or SEGs, for that matter) were the same in each District in the Region, controlling for supply in a study of social factors and use of services would still be difficult to achieve. The possibility cannot be excluded that the higher use observed in inner city areas is the product not of current high levels of supply, but conditioned by high levels of supply in the past. If this is so, it is impossible ever to correct data satisfactorily for supply, to arrive at a social factor weighting for "need".

Taking the analysis of utilisation and ACORN further, researchers at St Thomas's Hospital Medical School propose to investigate the relative resource requirements of hospital inpatients in different ACORN Groups by looking at the length of hospital stay of samples of patients with the same diagnosis and treatment (as identified by Diagnosis Related Groups), but from different ACORN Groups. It is planned to collect these data in a number of Districts with contrasting levels of health service provision. Through this research it is hoped to be able to identify ACORN Groups which place a particular burden on local health services and to observe the consistency (or otherwise) of the relationship between length of stay, social conditions and the availability of beds for similar cases. Consideration will be also given to including data on the quality of primary care: a potentially important influence on the demand for hospital care but one which has not hitherto been studied empirically.

The Jarman Index of 'Under-privileged Areas' and the Need for Primary Care Services

Approaches to developing needs weightings for RAWP using utilisation data tend to be dominated by the use of hospital services, since data are far more plentiful in this sector. Far less consideration has been given to specific indicators of the need for community health services. However, an entirely different approach to identifying the need for health care in different social areas based on the views of health care professionals has been pioneered for primary care and community health services by Jarman. Jarman's long-term objective was to develop a technique to guide the deployment of general practitioner services in relation to likely demand (not need) for their services. However, this method has been discussed as a possible alternative to the SMR as a measure of need in RAWP.

In analysing the evidence submitted to the Acheson Committee on primary care in London (London Health Planning Consortium, 1981) Jarman became aware of a strong consensus among those submitting evidence, that certain social characteristics were deemed to be associated with greater pressure on primary care services (eg. elderly living alone). Jarman corroborated the impressions of the London GPs with a national questionnaire survey which asked a 1 in 10 random sample of GPs in the United Kingdom to score each of a list of social factors on a scale from 0 (no problem) to 9 (very problematical) according to the degree to which each one was thought to increase his/her GP workload (Jarman, 1983). Census data relating to the social factors identified by the GPs has been used to calculate composite workload scores ('underprivileged areas scores') for all areas of England and Wales down to ward or Enumeration District level by adding the standardised values of each variable in each geographical area, weighted by the scores for each variable in the GP survey (Irving, 1983a).

The "Jarman Index" as it is known, defines areas by the concentration of social factors which GPs nationally have weighted according to the degree to which they increase their workload. Thus, it is a potential means for giving extra support to GPs in the areas where they may be under the greatest pressure due to the social characteristics of the communities they serve. Jarman has attempted to validate his results by administering the same questionnaire to a sample of community nurses in a District. This produced similar results to the GP survey. As a result the "Jarman Index" has been used by certain Health Districts to target community nursing manpower on small areas.

In addition, comparison between maps of the Jarman Index and maps of the Department of the Environment social deprivation index has shown a high degree of correspondence (Irving 1983b). As another form of validation, Jarman asked the Local Medical Committees in five FPC areas to shade blank ward maps according to the degree to which the populations increased GP workload or pressure on their services. These maps were then compared with maps of the calculated scores from the Jarman Index. Overall only 6.3% of the wards differed in any way (Jarman, 1984).

What are the implications of Jarman's work for resource allocation? The community health services component of the RAWP formula takes account of population size, age/sex structure and SMR. Jarman's co-worker, Irving, argues that this is inadequate. Firstly, it excludes the services of GPs and other independent contractors who are not funded by the RHAs and DHAs, but whose activities are a major determinant of hospital admissions and therefore of resource demands made on DHAs. Secondly, the age/sex and SMR adjustments do not necessarily compensate for the added difficulties of providing primary care services in declining urban areas. Thirdly, the formula is designed to calculate the total funding of DHAs and is not capable of drawing attention to areas below District level which may experience special difficulties (Irving, 1983a). Irving argues that the Jarman 'underprivileged area score' could be used to target community health services at local level and perhaps as an additional factor in resource allocation. However, is a score based on the opinion of GPs, in any sense an objective indicator of need? Jarman himself describes the index as suitable for planning the distribution of general practitioners, but recognises that it does not amount to a measure of "need" comparable to SMRs nor a measure of GP workload (Jarman, 1985).

Although Jarman himself has produced favourable results from validation studies of his Index using further GPs' and community nurses' perceptions (Jarman, 1983 and 1984), it is difficult to find independent need data for a proper validation of the potential of the Index as a genuine measure of need. However, Charlton and Lakhani (1985) compared the Jarman score firstly, with mortality from selected causes amenable to GP intervention and secondly with the incidence of two diseases (cervical cancer and tuberculosis) where GP intervention is important. Significant positive correlations indicated that the scores had some external criterion validity as a measure of "need" for GP services. The authors concluded that more detailed research would be required to establish its validity firmly enough for it to be used to achieve greater equity in the distribution of GP services and community health services.

This advice is reinforced by validation studies in Manchester which show that although high ward scores on the 'underprivileged area' index appeared in general to be associated with greater needs for health care as judged by mortality, low birth weight and prevalence of disability; contrary to expectations, the GPs in wards with the worst scores had the highest doctor:patient ratios, spent less time on average with their patients than GPs with surgeries in the best wards and were less likely to feel overworked than colleagues in other areas (Leavey and Wood, 1985). This would seem to indicate that the type and level of need in an area is not necessarily the main influence on a GP's workload and pressure of work. The organisation of general practice and the ability and motivation of the GP may be far more significant in translating socio-medical need into actual workload. Leavey and Wood have added an important dimension to the debate about the need for primary care services by drawing attention to features of the survices rather than the social environment.

It is frequently asserted that since primary care services, especially general practitioner services, are poor in needy inner city areas and the demand for hospital beds is much higher as a result, the problem is one of a lack of investment in inner city general practice. It is argued that one way to improve matters is to increase expenditure in these areas. Jarman favours using his index of 'underprivileged areas' to target such resources. However, the problem is complex. In fact, with only a few exceptions, FPC expenditure on General Medical Services appears to be positively correlated with the level of expenditure of the corresponding health authority expressed as its distance from RAWP target (Bevan and Charlton, 1986). Since the majority of the over-target health authorities are in the cities where the worst primary care is said to be, this raises interesting questions about what the appropriate distributive policy response should be.

To develop a response, it is important to get behind the raw data on rates of expenditure in relatively large administrative units (Bevan, 1985) and the superficial characteristics of general practice (eg. list sizes) (Leavey and Wood, 1985) to consider the effectiveness of delivery of primary care and its accessibility to patients. For example, it is likely that significant differences exist in the levels and quality of primary care available within different parts of any one city. Data from four Scottish cities in the mid-1970s suggested that GP surgeries tended to be concentrated in deprived inner city centres and in the longer established private residential areas with few in postwar peripheral areas (Knox, 1978). In terms of spatial accessibility (derived from a gravity model) the pattern tended to be one of a stark disparity between central and peripheral areas with the highest levels of accessibility in the older inner city areas which included both deprived and non-deprived parts. Beyond the inner core, accessibility was inversely related to socio-economic status. The worst served parts of the four cities were the large, deprived, peripheral public housing estates which would normally be associated with above-average rates of morbidity. In these estates car ownership was low and bus services infrequent.

These data lend only limited support to a strategy of channelling resources into multiply deprived inner city areas since the two extremes of deprivation (the inner city and the peripheral estates) emerged as best and worst-off respectively in accessibility to primary care. However, in terms of crude indicators of quality, rather than availability, the inner city areas emerged as worst-off with high proportions of elderly, single-handed practitioners working from inadequate premises, similar to the stereotype of general practice in inner London (Knox, 1979).

After a validation exercise, Jarman's Index of perceived workload pressure on primary care services was adopted by the BMA to identify wards it would regard as 'underprivileged' and so eligible for special help in improving services. A number of FPCs and community units in DHAs have used the method as an indicator of the need for a variety of community health services and analyses of District scores and values of the individual variables are now available on computer disc (Irving, 1985). The technique is regarded as useful for identifying localities for special programmes of community health services, since it is not affected by the administrative separation of DHAs and FPCs (Irving, 1983b).

Before the Jarman Index becomes NHS orthodoxy, it is timely to assess its limitations and the value of alternatives. Since Jarman's 'underprivileged area' score originated in a questionnaire drawn from an analysis of the written comments of GPs and health care organisations in London submitted to the Acheson Committee, it is possible that it is biased towards deprivation factors which are more common in the capital than elsewhere. The "worst" Districts in England according to the Jarman Index, tend to be in inner London. This constrasts with a number of other indices of deprivation. Two particular social variables stand out because of their Regional variation: the unemployment rate and the proportion of ethnic minorities in the population (eg. Mersey RHA has the highest unemployment but the lowest concentration of ethnic minorities and it is unclear what effect this has on the need for health services) (Irving, 1985).

In recognition of unemployment conditions on Merseyside an alternative approach to measuring the need for primary care which includes permanent sickness rates as well as other social variables has been developed in Mersey RHA and promulgated by Scott-Samuel (1984). Scott-Samuel has been deeply critical of Jarman's work and pointed out, among other things, that:

1. The 'underprivileged areas' score lacks objectivity since it is based entirely on the views of general practitioners (including the validation exercise by Local Medical Committees).

2. The social factors in the score were selected through a national survey of the views of GPs about factors identified previously by a very small percentage of London GPs who gave evidence to the Acheson Committee.

3. The allocation of resources should be based on the community's needs, not on the workload they are perceived to generate.

The objective measure of need which Scott-Samuel uses is the proportion of the population not in employment due to permanent sickness, as recorded in the Census. An index of need has been developed, based on this measure and incorporating ten Census social indicators which explain substantial proportions of the variance in permanent sickness between local authority areas in Mersey RHA, weighted according to their correlation with the sickness variable (Mersey Regional Health Authority, 1983). However, it is not immediately clear why, if permanent sickness rates are an objective indicator and are available for the whole country, it is necessary to derive a more complex indicator from correlated social variables rather than use the permanent sickness rate alone. Presumably Scott-Samuel wished to include elements which related to variations in the socio-economic environment which underline simple morbidity differences (Thunhurst, 1985).

The score for the permanent sickness measure was compared with the Jarman Index score for each of the wards in Liverpool. The two scores varied substantially.

In 19 of the 33 wards the Jarman score was higher than the score based on chronic sickness and related social conditions. Scott-Samuel concluded that the Jarman Index could not be thought of as a measure of health service "need".

By using Census data for both morbidity and social conditions, Scott-Samuel has produced an index of need which unlike SMRs, can be used down to ward and ED level. However, for RAWP-type resource allocation, this fine detail is not required. In fact, in the same Mersey RHA study which Scott-Samuel used to derive his 'objective indicator', the permanent sickness variable was found to correlate very highly with SMR at local authority District level. The conclusion once again was that the SMR was a good proxy for morbidity at DHA level and therefore, an SMR weighting in sub-Regional RAWP was reasonable. However, it was recognised that there might be other dimensions of morbidity not picked up by SMR, since there were a number of social variables closely correlated with permanent sickness but not with SMR (eg. male unemployment rate). These social variables were highly inter-correlated and any one could have been used as an additional RAWP weighting. Whether a further weighting was deemed necessary, the Mersey researchers sensibly concluded was a matter of judgement (Mersey Regional Health Authority, 1983).

RURAL DEPRIVATION AND SPARSITY OF POPULATION

Before leaving the question of how to allow for socio-economic conditions in NHS resource allocation, a few comments must be made about conditions in rural areas and their impact on access to and need for health care. Protagonists in the "social deprivation debate" have tended to assume a specifically urban notion of social deprivation and have conducted their discussions particularly around the fate of inner London populations served by historic, prestigious teaching hospitals. However, there are high SMRs and adverse social conditions to be found in rural as well as urban areas. Furthermore, by concentrating resources primarily in relation to population size, age and sex structure and morbidity it can be argued that RAWP excludes two important geographical factors found in rural areas, which are not strictly deprivation factors, namely:

1. The potential effect of geographical dispersion of population in increasing the costs of providing health care; for example, through longer inpatient stays for distant patients (Wood, 1984). If the resource allocation formula ignores these additional costs, territorial inequities will remain. The policy response in this case is to increase the overall level of resources to the health authority since the whole population has suffered a relative loss in its chances of obtaining medical care because the health authority's average cost of provision has been increased and it will obtain less health care per unit of expenditure.

2. The potential effect of distance as a barrier to access for some patients which may impede the attainment of equal access (Wood, 1984). Distant patients may under-utilise facilities in relation to need or incur greater costs than nearby patients. The policy response to this problem requires not only the provision of more resources but also a mechanism for ensuring that resources are directed to those who are disadvantaged.

Heller (1979) adds a third factor associated with rural areas, namely the poor quality of the facilities which are provided to widely dispersed populations as resoruces are increasingly centred on urban hospital complexes.

The RAWP report does not discuss the rural dimension or the possible effect of distance on costs and utilisation, although a weighting is given for the additional costs of employing staff in London. The ambulance component of the RAWP formula was designed without an allowance for the increased distances travelled in rural areas. By contrast the Scottish Health Authorities Revenue Equalisation (SHARE) report does include a 'sparsity factor' in the community health services component of the formula in recognition of the fact that large parts of some Health Boards are very thinly populated. The SHARE report states that it might be expected that a higher provision of community health services would be required in these areas because providers would have to spend more time travelling and would generally have to have a smaller caseload than in more densely populated areas. The 'sparsity factor' is based on an estimate of the proportion of a community nurse's time likely to be spent on travelling and on data available from the calculation of the Scottish Rural Practices Fund (mileage payments for country GPs) (Scottish Home and Health Department, 1977, p.15, para 3.20). The 'sparsity factor' in SHARE appears to be concerned with the public costs to the NHS of distance and sparsity of population and gives no attention to the costs to individual patients. It thus responds to the first of the geographical factors identified, but not the second. It is likely that the problem of compensating for the higher unit costs of provision in rural areas can be resolved at far less cost than the disadvantage suffered by individuals in remote locations.

The problems of gaining access to health facilities in rural areas do not impinge equally on all social groups. Heller (1979) maintains that those groups who are potentially most in need (eg. the elderly, women with young children, lower income groups) have the greatest problems of access. Using data from East Anglia he also estimates that provision per capita in rural areas is often far below the national average. Within the Region, expenditure is concentrated on urban areas and "centres of excellence" with commensurately lower provision in remote parts. All the rural health Districts in East Anglia had expenditure levels on both hospital and community health services in the 1970s far below the national average per capita. In these Districts, surgical waiting lists were much longer than in the urban Districts in the Region and a much higher proportion of the population had to travel outside the District for routine treatment.

While Heller (1979) has gathered statistical material on rural health deprivation in terms of the availability of resources, his analysis does suggest that a significant proportion of the population is prepared to travel outside rural Districts for treatment. The question arises as to the extent of the welfare losses which may be associated with the need to travel long distances for health care among those who do not receive treatment. Wood (1984) studied the effect of distance and population density on utilisation and length of stay for surgical inpatients in Grampian Region in Scotland, where hospital services and population are concentrated in Aberdeen, with an extensive, sparsely populated, rural hinterland. The conclusions of the study were that distance and sparsity factors represented only a minor source of territorial inequity, but that for specific groups within the population spatial inequalities in access might arise. For certain operations, length of stay was found to be related to distance of the patient's home from Aberdeen, but overall, this accounted for a very small part of the variations in length of stay and had minor resource implications. The analysis of utilisation rates suggested that it was sparsity of population and access to the GP rather than distance from the main medical centre which influenced access to hospital care, particularly for elderly patients. In total distance and sparsity effects accounted for very little of the observed variation in discharge rates and lengths of stay. Wood's overall conclusion is that the importance of spatial inequality associated with rural areas should not be overstated, particularly in comparison with social class inequalities in access. However, Wood's analysis does not include consideration of the relative private costs of utilisation incurred by people from different parts of the Region. Wood recognises in his discussion that inequalities of access may continue to exist even when levels of utilisation do not differ between areas, if individuals have to travel widely different distances. To overcome this aspect of inequality would require making funds available to health authorities so that they could compensate patients who have to travel long distances for treatment. All-in-all, it does not seem that sparsity of population in rural areas is a major factor for geographical resource allocation.

OVERVIEW: SMRs, SOCIAL INDICATORS AND THE NEED FOR HEALTH CARE

RAWP chose to weight the population using the SMR as a proxy for the differences in morbidity between geographical areas which remained when the age/sex composition of the population had been taken into account. In turn, morbidity was presumed to bear a direct relationship to the health care needs of a population. The relative need of a population was then translated into resource terms using utilisation data. RAWP was guided in this, firstly, by evidence that the available morbidity statistics, though imperfect, exhibited positive geographical correlations with mortality rates and, secondly, by the fact that mortality rates appeared to be the only available morbidity indictors which would meet the fairly stringent criteria required for inclusion in a resource allocation formula for the NHS. These criteria included, independence from the existing supply of resources, regular production, accuracy, availability at RHA and AHA level and a capacity to be broken down by age, sex and diagnosis. Thus, RAWP accepted mortality as a proxy for resource need because there were no other comprehensive, practicable, geographic morbidity measures available.

The initial response to RAWP's choice was to criticise the SMR as a surrogate for morbidity. These criticisms operated within RAWP's own, epidemiological definition of the need for health care resources as the prevalence and incidence of disease in a population. Under this definition it was assumed that morbidity would reflect the social, economic and environmental conditions of an area, since adverse conditions were known to increase susceptibility to death and disease. Thus, the two main criticisms levelled at the SMR were that it did not take adequate account of chronic disease and disability which burdened the Health Service, but resulted in few deaths; and that it did not always correlate sufficiently closely with the available morbidity data to be used as a morbidity proxy (Radical Statistics Health Group, 1977; Forster, 1977). However, latterly, the main body of criticism of the use of mortality data has shifted beyond the original RAWP definition of the need for health care. SMRs have come to be criticised for their incompleteness in not taking explicit account of the effects of social deprivation on need and the difficulty and extra cost of delivering services in deprived areas (Fox, 1978; Woods, 1982). The contest around the definition of need has progressed from "need as morbidity", to "need as morbidity, plus the impact of social conditions on meeting need". It is argued that social conditions in a locality can place extra demands (and therefore, extra needs) on the NHS for any given level of morbidity and that these needs cannot be adequately recognised in the value of the various morbidity measures available, particularly not measures of mortality. This chapter has detailed the arguments surrounding the second of the two definitions of need and shown how ever more indirect proxies for morbidity based on social indicators have found their way into sub-Regional RAWP procedures. These proxies are weighted to be used as measures of need by reference to patterns of utilisation. This makes it difficult to disentangle the hypothesised extra needs in deprived areas from effects generated by the higher than average level of resources. The use of these proxies rests on shaky theoretical, methodological and evidential foundations. The general approach to allowing for social factors beyond morbidity in RAWP has tended to rely on studies of the relationship of a range of social deprivation indicators to data on the use of various types of health services. Yet, it has long been recognised that hospitalisation rates cannot be used to measure morbidity. Thus, the main drawback with these analyses remains how to correct the results for the effect of supply on use, irrespective of need, since it seems reasonable to assume that utilisation rates mainly reflect availability and ease of access to beds. The problem has not been satisfactorily resolved in either the North Thames inpatient census or the South East Thames ACORN Study (North East Thames Regional Health Authority, 1983a and 1983b; South East Thames Regional Health Authority, 1985 and 1986a). It rears its head again in a recent attempt to relate admission rates to a range of "deprivation" indices, including ACORN and the Jarman index, in order to replace the SMR with a more sensitive indicator in RAWP (Butts, 1986). Hospital bed-use rates can only be used in studies of relatively restricted areas in which bed availability can be assumed to be equal. Thus, Carstairs (1981) was able to show in a study within Glasgow and Edinburgh where beds were effectively equally available, that populations near to hospitals had lower levels of use than more deprived populations further away. However, this still assumes that the existing pattern of use can be equated with need. Furthermore, to be useful for resource allocation, studies have to include areas with differing levels of supply!

Despite these problems, indicators of "social deprivation" identified by their association with patterns of use, are still seen as the way forward in sub-Regional RAWP in the Thames Regions. The NHS has neglected to develop systems for collecting better, direct, measures of morbidity such as through extending existing disease registers and using community morbidity surveys. A series of surveys could be used to look at the relationship between various aspects of morbidity and material and social characteristics of populations in a representative range of Districts; thus avoiding contamination by supply factors. The results could be used to give widely available social indicators (eg. from the national Census) an empirical morbidity weighting. In this way the social characteristics of all Districts could be employed to predict the likely mortality and morbidity experience of their populations and in turn their need for health care resources.

It is an interesting reflection on the nature of the debate about including social deprivation in RAWP that it has centred almost exclusively on the supposedly unique and highly complex needs of inner London. There has been little discussion outside the Thames Regions despite the existence of deprived inner city areas elsewhere. Similar gradients of mortality and morbidity exist between inner and outer zones in other cities and these tend to be highly correlated with measures of socio-economic deprivation. Indeed, the areas of highest mortality and morbidity and the worst material deprivation are overwhelmingly to be found in the North and North West, with the exception of one or two localities in inner London. Yet the case for inner London continues to be made vigorously. Balarajan (1986) recently contended that it was irrational to move resources out of inner London since inner London constituted the largest socially deprived area in the country. In response a group from Sheffield pointed out that when indicators such as the percentage of unemployed people, or of unskilled workers, were used to rank Districts, the inner London Districts fared very favourably compared with inner city Districts elsewhere (Milner, Johnson, Watts, et al, 1986). It follows from this that part of the conflict may stem from different definitions of what constitutes "deprivation". The case for special treatment for London tends to be made on the basis of factors such as the proportion of people in private rented accommodation and the proportion of New Commonwealth and Pakistan immigrants. These tend to be features of the capital. However, it is unclear to what extent such features are likely to be implicated in poor health. There has been a tendency to use measures of deprivation in order to argue a case against RAWP without considering the rationale behind the selection of the variables which went into the measure. In studying health and deprivation, Townsend, Phillimore and Beattie (1986, pp. 177-8) argue that material deprivation needs to be distinguished from <u>social</u> deprivation. By <u>material</u> deprivation, Townsend and colleagues mean the lack of goods, services, resources, amenities and physical environment which are customary in a society and which in turn, are known to have an adverse effect on health (eg. poverty). Furthermore, a distinction needs to be drawn between direct experience of deprivation and membership of a sub-group or minority at risk of that aspect of deprivation. Thus, the proportion of New Commonwealth immigrants in an area would not be regarded as a suitable measure of deprivation by Townsend <u>et al</u> on the grounds that it does not give direct information about the material conditions of the immigrant group. It is worth quoting their justification for this view at length:

'It is we believe mistaken to treat being black, or old and alone, or single parenthood as part of the definition of deprivation. Even if many among these minorities <u>are</u> deprived, some are not and the point is to find out how many are <u>deprived</u> rather than operate as if all were in that condition. It is the form their deprivation takes and not their status which has to be measured.'
(Townsend, Phillimore and Beattie, 1986, p.48)

The choice of indicators is important in determining the ranking of Districts according to levels of deprivation and this, in turn, can influence the debate about RAWP and social deprivation. Variables which relate to minorities at risk of deprivation, such as single parenthood and ethnicity, tend to give high deprivation scores for a number of inner London Boroughs and relatively low scores for Northern and Western parts of the country. For example, the index of 'underprivileged areas' developed by Jarman, locates seven of the ten most deprived Districts in England in London, but none in the Northern Region (Jarman, 1984). Five of the eight variables in the Jarman index merely reflect minorities potentially at risk of deprivation. Similarly, Balarajan (1986) bases his case for reversing RAWP redistribution to favour inner London on the basis of factors such as the proportion of immigrants and elderly people living alone and a general argument that the extent of multiple deprivation in inner London is 'unqiue' and complex. By contrast, Townsend's index of material deprivation used to study the relationship between ill-health and deprivation in the Northern Region consists of four measures chosen specifically to reflect the extent to which populations are likely to have direct experience of material deprivation adversely affecting health:

1. unemployment as a measure of a general lack of material resources and insecurity;

2. car ownership as a surrogate for current income;

3. home ownership as a reflection of a lack of wealth as well as income;

4. overcrowding as an indicator of poor housing.
   (Townsend, Phillimore and Beattie, 1986, pp. 48-51)

The most deprived areas using these measures of material circumstances tend to be in the North and West of England.

Despite the continuing pressure for an additional social deprivation weighting in sub-Regional RAWP in the Thames Regions, the literature tends to show a high degree of correlation between mortality, morbidity and adverse social and environmental factors at DHA level and even below (Brennan and Lancashire, 1978; Knox, Marshall, Kane, Green and Mallett, 1980; Townsend, Simpson and Tibbs, 1984; Townsend, Phillimore and Beattie, 1986). This raises doubts about whether it is justifiable to include a weighting for social deprivation in the formula which is essentially about the comparative need for health care defined in terms of relative morbidity. Carstairs (1982) completed her review of the relationship between health and social deprivation by stating that:

> '... the upward gradients which have been shown in both hospital use and the SMR with increasing deprivation provide some support for the use of the SMR as a good overall measure of need in the resource allocation formulae, ...'

RAWP's choice of mortality data has been criticised on the grounds that mortality (and morbidity) are "downstream" indicators in that they do not identify the underlying social conditions responsible for inequalities in health. It is argued that the focus must move "upstream" (Thunhurst, 1985). Yet the case for using mortality data is strengthened by reflecting on the direction of causality in the relationship between deprivation, morbidity and mortality. Although by no means all morbidity and mortality is the direct result of deprivation, the direction of causality is <u>from</u> deprivation <u>to</u> morbidity and mortality. Thus, the mortality experience of a population is the product of the complex interaction of all the demographic, cultural, social, material and environmental factors acting upon that population. In this sense, mortality encapsulates a wider range of "deprivation" variables than any single measure of deprivation could do. For example, there is evidence that mortality rates demonstrate the impact not only of demographic and socio-economic differences between different Regions of England, but also environmental differences which affect health. Thus, mortality rates in the North and West of the country are consistently higher than those in the South East even when demographic and socio-economic variations are allowed for. Social class standardisation has almost no relative effect on the Regional all-cause SMRs nor on Regional infant mortality rates (Office of Population Censuses and Surveys, 1978). It appears that area of residence is an independent variable affecting health. A similar variation in mean systolic and diastolic blood pressure has been observed between towns in the South East and North of Great Britain, independent of age, body mass index, alcohol use, smoking, social class and marital status (McIntyre, 1986). The OPCS longitudinal study also provides evidence which suggests that geographical variations in mortality are, at least in part, the product of an interaction between socio-economic status and environmental variables (Fox, Jones and Goldblatt, 1984). It may be that the level of atmospheric pollution in the present, or at an earlier period, contributes to these findings. Townsend, Phillimore and Beattie (1986) encountered mortality variations between towns in the North East which could not be explained statistically by demographic, social, or material factors. The conclusion of such analyses for this discussion would appear to be that mortality (or morbidity) data have the advantage of reflecting a wider range of conditions which the NHS will have to respond to in an area, than a more restricted measure of social deprivation could encompass. The SMR is therefore to be preferred for general resource allocation.

The evidence would appear to support Carstairs' conclusion that mortality is a good measure of the need for health care resources, defined in terms of the level of morbidity in a population produced by the environmental, social, cultural and material circumstances of the population (Carstairs, 1982). However, it is still theoretically possible to argue a case for the recognition of needs in RAWP which are neither the consequence of morbidity nor of material deprivation, but simply of cultural and social "differentness" between areas. A good example is the challenge created for the NHS by the presence of ethnic minority communities. Their current needs in health service terms are unlikely to be reflected fully either in mortality data or in indicators of material deprivation, but in a combination of both, together with evidence about the extent to which meeting their needs imposes additional costs on local health services (eg. for interpreters). However, at present we lack good evidence that the presence of ethnic minorities does in fact, add significantly to NHS costs.

For example, certain ethnic minority groups have mortality rates for common causes substantially below the national average (Marmot, Adelstein and Bulusu, 1984). Much depends on the sensitivity of local management to the needs of minority groups. Studies are required to look at the problems and additional needs encountered by the NHS in its day-to-day operation as a result of specific social and cultural conditions in its working environment. The argument cannot remain at an anecdotal level. Investigations should be mounted, for example, to see whether patients in socially deprived Districts stay longer in hospital when case-mix is controlled for than would be expected by statistics of national average performance and why. Currently this sort of detailed evidence is lacking.

The use of social factors as proxies for morbidity and of the need for health care raises the question of whether a health services resource allocation formula should have built into it a wide range of social factors external to health services and to definitions of "health". Carstairs (1982) was unequivocal on this, 'Health need not deprivation, should provide the basis for determining health service delivery'. Social indicators are a far more indirect measure of morbidity than SMR. Their appropriateness is further challenged by the fact that most studies of health and deprivation conclude that the vast majority of the remedies for the differences observed in health and material conditions between deprived and non-deprived areas lie with wider social and economic programmes and not with curative or even preventive health services (Carlos, Martini, Allen, Davison and Backet, 1977). Seen in this light, allowances for social conditions in health service resource allocation should be designed so that they are for services which have a reasonable likelihood of improving the well-being of the deprived and of reaching the deprived themselves. The current tendency in sub-Regional RAWP is for the Thames Regions to replace the SMR with a global weighting for morbidity and social deprivation in one. This weighting results in an increment to the relevant Districts' general allocations to be spent on any service. In inner London this usually means a reduction in the distance over-target of teaching Districts. The deprived people in the District may not benefit at all from the additional funds they have caused to be retained, since the money may be used to support highly specialised services serving a national or Regional catchment (Haywood and Yates, 1986).

The debate about RAWP and social deprivation leads directly to the wider question of how to define the "need" for health care. The RAWP approach was based on a desire to put the measurement of need on a rational, objective basis. RAWP chose to define need in terms of morbidity. Evaluative judgement was to be limited to the initial choice of the indicators of "need as morbidity" after which, factual evidence would drive the resource allocation process. Thus RAWP expressed no requirement that the health care provided from the financial resources made available, be effective. RAWP's definition also avoided any reference to potentially controversial judgements about the objectives of the NHS. The way in which resources were used was a matter for health authorities to decide with reference to national guidance. Much of the literature criticising the SMR has focused similarly on the technical selection of the "right" indicator, the quality of the data sources, the impact on targets of changes in the indicators and so on. The SMR stands up to much of this criticism fairly well. However, the debate is bound to remain inconclusive since implicit even in the technical criticisms of the RAWP approach, are rival judgements about how needs hould be defined and which needs should be funded and which not. Yet there is no agreed "objective" basis for determining the need for health services. Thus, the criticism of the SMR for being an incomplete proxy for the need for health care because it does not make allowance for social conditions implies a wider role for the Health Service in combating adverse social conditions than has been customary hitherto and therefore, an enlarged definition of the need for health care. This immediately calls for judgement as to the wisdom of extending the NHS' remit. By contrast, RAWP's pragmatic definition of need had the virtue of avoiding the need for this sort of policy decision. It is highly unlikely that a societal consensus can easily be reached as to the "right" balance between NHS objectives of prevention, cure and care. Since 1976, a number of writers have tried to sharpen the focus of RAWP's pragmatic definition. Thus Acheson (1978) proposed a definition based on medical expertise and health care evaluation. He argued that need for health care should be defined by whether or not there was judged to be an appropriate and effective medical treatement or response. Snaith (1978) adopted a similar approach based on evaluations and clinical trials. The 'worth' of a service or range of services should be evaluated and on the basis of proven benefits, decisions should be taken on how much to provide and where. In the same vein, Patrick, Holland, Palmer and West (1980) gave a definition of the need for health care which related resource allocation to planning. In their view the need for health care for resource allocation purposes was best defined by the preventive, curative and caring, objectives of the NHS. This would entail explicit value judgements to be made about the relative importance of these three main functions of the health sector. They commented, 'Only by stating clearly what the Health Service is supposed to be doing can we identify those aspects of ill-health which warrant resource provision and develop data collection systems and statistical methods for measuring resource needs'. Under this sort of approach, measures of resource need relevant to objectives and priorities (ie. mortality or morbidity data for conditions or diseases which were preventable, curable or required care which the NHS was able to give) could then be linked to current and projected spending patterns (Palmer, 1978, p.35). Brennan and Clare (1980) proposed a similar integrated approach to resource allocation and planning in which allocations were to be determined by long-term priorities. Under such a system, mortality data would be incorporated into the planning indicators used to determine the relative need for particular services in different areas.

The basic assumption behind Patrick et al (1980) and Brennan and Clare (1980) is that the allocation of resources to particular aspects of need should reflect not only the prevalence of disease, but also (and more importantly) the relative priority attached by society, decision-makers, health care providers and others to meeting those needs. This requires that objectives for the NHS should be clearly articulated: that the balance between prevention, care and cure and between services for children, the elderly, the mentally ill, and other groups should be publicly established, in line with prevailing social and cultural values. Once this has been accomplished, it is argued, a variety of indicators of the need for resources different from those in the conventional RAWP formula can be selected.

An approach to need based on explicit societal objectives and priorities rather than those implicit in the often contradictory pattern of much current Health Service activity is intellectually attractive. However, it presumes that a consensus will emerge from the views and priorities of a wide range of different groups rather than conflicts of values and interests. It also assumes that society is willing to make the difficult choices in health care explicit. It is doubtful if either of these is likely to be the case. In these circumstances, the great attraction of the RAWP approach was that it appeared to skirt difficult issues about NHS objectives and priorities. However, the conflict over objectives did not disappear because it was ignored or made implicit. One way of interpreting "the RAWP and social deprivation debate" is in terms of rival definitions of the need for health care, which in turn, reflect different priorities for the NHS and health policy in general. Thus if the view is that the Health Service should be responsive to the needs produced by the social conditions under which it operates, regardless of its ability fundamentally to alter their causes, then it would seem appropriate to include social weightings in resource allocation formulae. By contrast, if the main concern is to ensure that the NHS deals with those medical aspects of health and disease which it is capable of affecting, while the main social, economic and lifestyle determinants of disease are tackled directly by other agencies, then it would seem appropriate to restrict the NHS resource allocation formulae to morbidity weightings. Unfortunately, the remit of the NHS has never been precisely defined and in reality it is difficult to make a clear distinction between the medical and the social function (Klein, 1977).

The "RAWP and social deprivation debate" can also be understood in political terms. Since RAWP concerns the sharing out of scarce resources, it cannot avoid being a source of political controversy within the NHS and to a lesser extent outside. This is irrespective of debates over the "right" definition of the need for health care resources. Regions have been faced with the problem of securing voluntary agreement from the "losers" to a process of reallocation in the face of many unkowns about the measurement of need for health care resources (Walker, 1978). One way of doing this in the Thames Regions, where historic inequalities in resource availability were greatest and therefore, controversy over redistribution was fiercest, was to include an allowance for social conditions in sub-Regional RAWP. Resource allocation remains a political issue in which decisions have to be taken on the basis of imperfect knowledge with a view either to retaining the historically unequal status quo, or changing it in the direction of some notion of equity. There is a grave danger that the emphasis given to the debate over the SMR in the literature exaggerates the relative importance of factors other than the age/sex structure and overall size of populations in determining their relative need for health service resources. The scale of variation in the RAWP-weighted per capita availability and consumption of health resources between Districts in the NHS is still huge as recent DHSS Performance Indicators have shown (DHSS, 1985a and 1986b). Seen in this perspective, the choice of additional need weightings over and above population size and age/sex structure, such as SMRs, social deprivation or ACORN, are of secondary importance compared with ensuring that NHS resource allocation continues to move towards overcoming the grossest differences between different parts of the country. The debate about the measurement of need for health care resources will continue in epidemiology and social science and it is right that it should. However, the uncertainties about, for example, whether the health needs of residents of inner city teaching Districts are adequately reflected in sub-Regional RAWP formulae should not paralyse the process of redistribution. Clearly, better morbidity and social deprivation data are required as Districts approach an equal distribution of services. However, these adjustments amount to fine-tuning the system compared to overcoming the fundamental inequalities in resource availability and utilisation which still exist between different Districts.

POSSIBLE WAYS FORWARD

National RAWP

For the allocation of funds by DHSS to RHAs the issue of choosing a morbidity weighting apart from the age/sex structure of the population is relatively less important than sub-Regionally, since RHAs are reasonably socially homogeneous and population size and age/sex structure dominate targets. The requirement at the level of setting RHA targets is for a simple weighting which distinguishes consistently between RHAs. Age-specific mortality ratios (ASMRs), perhaps supplemented by data on common chronic conditions which are known to vary in their incidence between different parts of the country would seem the best choice. The use of mortality data after the age/sex structures of populations have been accounted for, can be justified at this level for the following reasons:

1. In general, mortality data are highly correlated with the available measures of morbidity for the majority of diseases.

2. There appears to be little geographic variation in the prevalence of conditions for which mortality is a poor proxy of the need for health care resources.

3. Mortality data tend to be highly correlated with social factors associated with the need for health care.

4. Mortality is the most direct measure of the need for health care currently available, until investment is made in collection of better and more comprehensive morbidity data.

Sub-Regional RAWP

Sub-Regionally, the situation is more difficult, although the solution does not appear to lie in ever more refined variants of the RAWP formula especially not in the case of acute hospital services, but rather in the integration of resource allocation with planning through Regional strategic management (see Chapter Seven, 'RAWP and Planning', for a fuller discussion of this).

The precise approach depends on how resource allocation is pursued in each Region. Whichever method is chosen, objective measures of the need for health care will still be required to help guide managers towards an equitable distribution of services. The general approach will require the elaboration of the available morbidity measures and investment in special data collection. Nevertheless, unfashionable mortality data have been shown to be highly correlated with available morbidity and deprivation indices even at ward level and are capable of playing a major part in planning-led resource allocation (Brennan and Clare, 1980; Townsend, Phillimore and Beattie, 1986). It would only seem justifiable to stop using mortality data for planning and resource allocation when comprehensive disease registers covering a wide range of important conditions and regular community morbidity surveys are in place.

Under regional strategic management of sub-Regional equity, plans would be assessed and the likely effect of their implementation evaluated by the RHA according to whether or not they promoted movement towards an equitable distribution and utilisation of services. Under this approach, a variety of different sources of morbidity data with specific relevance to different services could be used when they become available in the future, rather than a monolithic definition of need as in the RAWP formula. Instead of monitoring progress towards an administrative target with the limited goal of securing an equitable distribution of financial inputs, the focus would be on ensuring that health services were both made available equitably and more importantly, utilised equitably in relation to various relevant measures of need.

With an integrated approach to planning and resource allocation, it should be possible to ensure that funds allocated to a District on the basis of an assessment of a particular set of needs are actually deployed in ways which informed opinion suggests have some relevance to meeting those same needs. This would help clarify the woolly thinking surrounding the needs of "socially deprived areas" for NHS resources. The current position (particularly in the Thames Regions) risks providing extra NHS resources to the inner city Districts on the evidence of various analyses of the relationship between social indicators and health service utilisation (there is still a major problem in adequately allowing for supply effects) without any assurance either that extra

Health Service resources are particularly relevant to the presumed needs of
these Districts, or that even if they are, they will actually be used to serve
those needs.

Many of todays's enthusiasts for the inclusion of social deprivation weightings
in sub-Regional RAWP would be more lukewarm if they had to show how the extra
resources they gained were to be used to, say, improve the health status of the
inner city population, rather than to bolster the existing pattern of
predominantly acute, hospital, services. Spending more on health services in
socially disadvantaged areas appears at first sight to be commonsense. Since
expenditure on health services is usually strongly supported in all sectors of
society, it is a politically attractive way of responding to urban social
deprivation. Yet the question remains as to whether it is the most effective
response to health need generated through socio-economic conditions which have
their origins far outside the control of the NHS.

PART TWO

USING RAWP TARGETS TO ACHIEVE EQUITY

CHAPTER SIX

MANAGING CROSS-BOUNDARY FLOWS OF PATIENTS
AND THE PURSUIT OF EQUITY

ALTERNATIVES TO CATCHMENT POPULATIONS FOR ACUTE SERVICES

In Chapter Three the problems inherent in the original RAWP method of estimating the extent of patient flows across boundaries and adjusting resident populations accordingly were discussed. Alternative methods of calculating catchment populations developed by a number of Regions to improve on RAWP, were also found wanting, since they embody unrealistic assumptions about future patterns of flows in a situation of progressive redistribution. A number of proposals have been put forward to circumvent these difficulties and thereby to abolish what Bevan (1986) calls the 'metaphysical abstraction' of catchment populations altogether. They are as follows:

1. to model future flows as part of a planning-led approach to resource allocation (Bevan, Beech and Craig, 1985)(see Chapter Seven);

2. to achieve equitable access to services by improving patient accessibility to the existing pattern of services rather than allocating equitable shares of finance to geographical populations (Dudley, 1977; Royal Commission on the National Health Service, 1978b);

3. to remove all flow adjustments from RAWP as part of a deliberate policy of fostering District autonomy (McCarthy, 1986) or as part of a quasi-market solution to the distribution of services in the NHS (Enthoven, 1985a);

4. to draw redraw health authority boundaries.

These remedies will be dealt with briefly in turn. With the exception of boundary revision, each represents an attempt to intervene in the processes which generate flows and therefore, in clinical freedom, where RAWP chose to accept flows as immutable "facts of life".

Modelling Future Flows

We lack good, empirical knowledge of the effect of large reductions in hospital capacity on patient flows although we have some data on the impact of opening new facilities. For example, the London Health Planning Consortium described the pattern of flows and utilisation rates before and after the opening of Northwick Park Hospital in Harrow (LHPC, 1979). However, when inequalities in resources have to be remedied in a phased manner, as under RAWP, one potentially productive approach would seem to lie with methods which enable health authorities to make informed <u>predictions</u> about the effect of movement to target on flows, rather than with the application of mechanistic catchment population methodologies. Bevan, Beech and Craig (1985) suggest that planning models could be used to predict the impact of the redistribution of revenue on cross-boundary flows and case-mix. Models would be revised from year-to-year in the light of the actual changes in flows brought about by the implementation of plans to change the distribution of services in line with equity. They entitle the approach Regional strategic management of equity and under it Regions would be encouraged to predict the impact on patient flows and utilisation rates of a sequence of changes in the distribution of resources and services (eg. through alterations in the capacity of individual hospitals) aimed at securing an equitable pattern of consumption across each Region. Existing flows would be assessed to see if they were reasonable or the product of inadequate facilities in certain Districts. Each District would negotiate phased changes in its services with its RHA and the finance it received would be based on planned, future numbers of beds and cases, assuming predetermined levels of efficiency. Thus, under regional strategic management of equity, DHA boundaries would have no role to play in the determination of allocations for acute services which would be based on an estimate of an equitable workload and there would be no need to estimate catchment populations (Bevan, Beech and Craig, 1985). There would thus be no direct link between Districts' allocations and their populations, rather an equitable Regional strategy for changing the distribution of services would act as the integrating element. Regional strategic management represents an attempt to coalesce the processes of resource allocation (RAWP) and planning and is discussed in this context in Chapter Seven, 'RAWP and Planning'.

Improving Patient Access to Existing Services

While regional strategic management entails planning future flows, the approach discussed by Dudley (1977) and Buxton and Klein (Royal Commission on the NHS, 1978b) takes RAWP's acceptance of the existing pattern of flows one stage further by proposing that access should be equalised by improving the mobility and information of patients and their referring doctors, rather than by simple, geographical, redistribution of services. This might involve such things as better transport, subsidised travel and information about waiting times and spare capacity. It would certainly involve leaving substantial cross-boundary flows in place and increasing them in specific contexts. Dudley (1977) sees this as a relatively quick way of getting patients to the hospitals which have the resources available to treat them compared with RAWP redistribution and one which avoids the destruction of existing clinical teams and facilities which it may not be straightforward to reconstitute elsewhere. He sees the approach as a logical extension of the concept of providing protected funding outside RAWP for Regional specialties, etc.. The approach has its attractions, particularly as a means of making a productive and more equitable use of the huge investment over the years in London which has resulted today in over-provision of acute services in relation to population, as defined by RAWP.

Buxton and Klein admit that it is not known how feasible such a scheme would be and what impact it would have on the well-known "distance decay effect" visible in current patterns of use of health services. It is not known how socially acceptable it would be, particularly for services other than short-stay surgery and it seems likely that even if the general approach were accepted, certain facilities would have to be physically relocated. In areas traditionally deprived in NHS terms, Dudley's vision would mean that clinicians would remain permanently dependent on the major centres of medical activity such as the metropolitan teaching hospitals for the care of their patients. The political attractiveness of such a scheme would seem to lie in the fact that it would avoid the embarassment of having to close hospitals in poor inner city areas and would protect "centres of excellence".

Dudley's approach begs the question of how clinician behaviour could be regulated to ensure fair access to the services by patients from peripheral

DHAs. How much freedom to make referrals would GPs and consultants in under-resourced Districts have? Equally, how would clinicians and managers in the Districts which are well-endowed be able to prioritise patients to ensure an equitable pattern of use? Would it be possible to use District of residence to decide who to treat? Furthermore, under Dudley's scheme the existing number of beds would remain in the over-target Districts and thus, there is a danger that local GPs would continue to refer at the same rates as in the past, squeezing out patients referred from further afield.

Under the sort of system envisaged by Dudley (1977), deprived Districts would be effectively "buying" services for their residents from Districts with the capacity to provide extra services so that maximum use would be made of the existing supply. However, he does not appear to envisage any formal charging mechanism being set up in recognition of this activity, rather the existing hospitals would be funded at cost for the work they did. However, more recent discussions of ways of equalising consumption of services without excessive physical redistribution and avoiding the need to calculate catchments, envisage explicit arrangements in which "deprived" Districts "buy" services from DHAs with excess capacity. This method is known as cross-charging and can take a wide range of forms. Enthoven (1985a) advocates a system in which Districts would be given the RAWP-weighted residential component of their target which they could either use to provide all the services they needed themselves, or to buy services for their residents from other Districts or the private sector. Districts would pay for emergency services at a standard cost and negotiate the price for other services competitively. In such a system, according to Enthoven, Districts would have incentives to seek high quality, cost-effective, health service suppliers for their residents and at the same time seek to provide good quality, cost-effective, services themselves to attract patients from other Districts and maximise income.

Cross-Charging

Whereas under RAWP, District managers have no control over their residents' use of services outside the District, cross-charging gives Districts the power to choose where their residents may be treated, since Districts will only pay for the treatment of their residents in other health authorities when this has been the subject of a specific contract. Since the contract is likely to give full details of the services to be provided at agreed costs and volumes, all cross-boundary flows for non-emergency cases will be controllable, predictable and accounted for, thus obviating the need for the estimation of catchment populations. At present cross-charging remains untried in the National Health Service with the exception of a few, small schemes related to hightly specific services (eg. provision of pacemakers). However it poses a number of major problems, among others, those of costing, freedom of referral, competition, emergency cases and rationing, which are discussed later in this chapter and in more detail in Brazier (1986) and Bevan (1986).

The general approach of giving Districts a fair share of revenue (for example, the RAWP residential component of their target) and the power to control residents' use of services outside the District has also been advocated by McCarthy (1986), but with a very different set of objectives in mind. Unlike Enthoven (1985a), whose goal is an 'internal market' in which DHAs and the private sector compete to provide the best and cheapest services, McCarthy wishes to construct a system in which allocations can be related to specific residential populations and District strategies to improve health can be easily evaluated against the resources committed to them. In practical terms, the compensation for cross-boundary flows would be removed from District RAWP targets and each authority would be given the RAWP-weighted residential component of its target and a clear responsibility for the resident population. Each District would be free to decide the blend of treatment, care and prevention it wished to provide from its resources and could be monitored according to its results. Cross-boundary flows could still exist, but they would be the result of planned agreements between Districts and directly controllable by the sending authority. Direct control over residents' use of services is a fundamental feature of both McCarthy's and Enthoven's proposals and can thus be seen as a potential solution to the problems of estimating catchment populations, encountered in conventional RAWP. However, McCarthy's use of resident populations as a basis for RAWP targets, with authorities being given explicit control over and responsibility for, services to their residents, has drawbacks, such as the requirement to interfere in clinical freedom of referral, similar in kind to Enthoven's proposals. These are discussed in greater detail in the section, 'Costing Cross-Boundary Flows' later in this Chapter and particularly in Brazier (1986) and Bevan (1986).

Boundary Changes

The final, commonsense option for dealing with cross-boundary flows in resource allocation is to redraw health authority boundaries to reduce the extent of flows. DHA boundaries, particularly in the conurbations, rarely match the natural catchments of hospitals for acute services. They were delineated to serve other purposes such as coterminosity with local authority areas for the provision of community services. Although boundary redrawing would probably reduce the extent of flows, it cannot eliminate flows altogether, particularly not in those parts of cities where their estimation is most problematic in RAWP. For example, it has been calculated that in 11 of the 59 Districts in the four Thames Regions 50% or more of the patients treated in the District are from other Districts and 50% or more of District residents are treated outside the District of residence (Brazier, 1986, personal communication). Changing boundaries is a palliative rather than a solution since it does not tackle the issue of how better to cope with adjustments to residential populations for cross-boundary flows. It merely reduces the extent of flows. Furthermore, it risks sacrificing the benefits of coterminosity where these exist and is likely to be unpopular in a Health Service weary of successive reorganisations and management changes.

DEALING WITH CROSS-BOUNDARY FLOWS OF OUTPATIENTS AND DAY CASES

Whichever of the above possible solutions to the problem of estimating cross-boundary flows for resource allocation is to be preferred, it is clear that the omission of any compensation for day, outpatient and accident and emergency cross-boundary flows in the original RAWP methods was a notable weakness. RAWP lacked adequate data on day and outpatient flows despite the fact that the day and outpatient component of the formula is generally second only to the non-psychiatric inpatient (NPIP) component in its contribution to the final target. Unlike SHARE in Scotland (Scottish Home and Health Department, 1977) RAWP chose not to use inpatient flows as a proxy measure for day and outpatients and did not assume that the pattern of inpatient flows corresponded with outpatient flows. There was evidence available to RAWP that the two sets of flows did not reliably mirror one another in many parts of the country (DHSS, 1976c, p.23, para. 2.18.3). Instead RAWP recommended as a matter of urgency that better information about these patients should be collected, particularly since they comprised a substantial and growing proportion of NHS expenditure. Agency arrangements could and should be taken into account.

After 1976 a number of relatively small-scale Regional studies of outpatient and day case flows took place, but their limited results did not amount to a basis for standard adjustments to the target for day and outpatients between Regions in national RAWP. The need still exists for a large-scale, national study

(Jones and Prowle, 1984, p.27). The same applies to flows of cases to accident and emergency departments. Currently, some Regions are attempting to include an allowance for day and outpatient cross-boundary flows in their own sub-Regional RAWP methods, but are handicapped by the lack of routine data. It is particularly difficult to trace these flows when they cross Regional boundaries (Brazier, 1986).

Beyond administrative neatness, why should it be important to include an allowance for day and outpatient flows in RAWP? What practical difference does its absence make? Theoretically, the lack of an allowance for day and outpatients risks creating perverse incentives against the development, where appropriate, of day care or outpatient treatment of cases currently treated as inpatients. DHSS has been seeking to encourage this development for some time (Royal Commission on the National Health Service, 1978b). This is because an authority receives no credit in its target for any inflows of day and outpatient cases. Although it seems unlikely that Districts have actually responded to these incentives in their planning or practice hitherto, with increasing financial pressure on the most over-target Districts, it may be only a matter of time before management is forced to consider the financial consequences of the so-called "good practice" of encouraging day surgery.

In more immediately practical terms, the lack of an allowance for day and outpatient flows has been regarded as unfairly penalising particular parts of the country. In general, at Regional level, commentators have pointed out that the accurate measurement of the extent (and cost) of these flows has little impact on targets. However, sub-Regionally it may be more important. For example, it has been of special concern in London since not only are there considerable inpatient flows in the capital, but the rate of outpatient attendance per 1000 resident population is much higher in London than the national average and accounts for a higher proportion of expenditure (Thompson and Lally, 1980, pp. 50-51; Greater London Council Health Panel, 1984, p.19). It is argued that non-residents are likely to be a significant element in these figures, coming into Central London for treatment but they are not picked up in RAWP calculations. On the other hand, it has to be realised that accounting for outpatient and day case cross-boundary flows may in fact make very little difference to inner London DHA targets as high inflows are often offset by high outflows to neighbouring Districts.

Worried by the lack of any compensation for London authorities and assuming that inflows out-numbered outflows, Senn and Shaw (1978) tested the effect of allocating expenditure on outpatient services within South East Thames RHA, according to either resident population or acute inpatient catchment populations (equivalent to resident populations adjusted by the Net Flow method). They found almost no correlation between resident populations of Districts and outpatient attendance rates, indicating either huge local variations in outpatient usage or extensive outpatient cross-boundary flows. The correlation of outpatient attendances with inpatient catchments was considerably higher. From this analysis, they concluded that in South East Thames at least, it would be possible to allocate day and outpatient resources for RAWP purposes using inpatient catchments in the manner of SHARE. Although South East Thames did not take up Senn and Shaw's suggestion, Trent Region was prepared to make an allowance in sub-Regional RAWP for outpatient flows in the absence of any data. Outpatient flow allowances were set arbitrarily at 50% of known inpatient flows (Holmes, 1984).

Other Regions have undertaken ad hoc surveys of outpatient flows between Districts. For example, North Western RHA surveyed the District of origin of 200,000 outpatient attendances over a four-week period in 1978 (Cottrell, 1979b). To test the adequacy of its rule-of-thumb allowance for outpatient flows, Trent RHA carried out a subsequent survey of outpatients by age, sex, specialty and place of residence over a two-week period in 1983. It found that in the main acute specialties, accounting for 75% of outpatients, the differences between the inpatient and outpatient served catchment populations were small: no more than 3% on average and easily explicable in each case. The Region was left with two options for modifying its RAWP formula: either to assume that inpatient and outpatient flows were identical for all practical purposes and to use HAA data to adjust for both sets of flows; or to use actual outpatient flow data from the survey in RAWP and consider regularly updating the results. The latter course of action exposed the limitations of the survey which for logistical reasons had only extended for a fortnight.

Over the years since 1976, Regional outpatient surveys have been ad hoc exercises over short time periods. Even within Regions they have rarely been adequate for making adjustments to sub-Regional RAWP because of the problem of flows to and from other Regions which are very substantial in the Thames Regions. For example, South East Thames RHA undertook a survey of outpatients and accident and emergency (A & E) cases, recording place of residence and place of treatment in order to be able to make adjustments to District targets for cross-boundary flows in these categories. Unfortunately, data were not available for out-flows to other Regions. Flows into South West Thames RHA from inner London Districts in South East Thames are particularly important for a true picture of where patients receive treatment. When the successor to RAWP, the Advisory Group on Resource Allocation, reported in 1980, it concluded that adequate data were still lacking and that a large-scale, national survey was required to enable consistent, empirical adjustments to be made for both national RAWP and sub-Regional variants (DHSS, 1980b, p.20). No action has been taken at national level on this since. AGRA also recommended that a start could be made by making adjustments to targets for cross-boundary flows of outpatients for kidney dialysis because the data were already available. This could be extended to other expensive outpatient services as data became available. Again no action has been taken to implement these recommendations. Currently, in most NHS Regions there are not even arbitrary adjustments for outpatient and day case cross-boundary flows in the manner of Trent RHA.

However, expedients do exist, if the prospect of regular Regional outpatient surveys is too daunting. North West Thames RHA has chosen to use a method for recognising day and outpatients for resource allocation similar to the original RAWP recommendations for long-stay mental illness patients, where, again, data on patient origin were lacking. For each District, the total number of expected outpatient and A & E attendances (calculated by applying national utilisation rates to DHA populations) is compared with the total of actual attendances (including residents and flows). The variance of actual to expected attendances is then deemed to be the net inflow or outflow and costed at the national average rate per attendance (North West Thames Regional Health Authority, 1984b).

The omission of a proper allowance for day and outpatient flows is likely to be far more significant in its impact on targets than the oft-discussed problem of whether RAWP methods adequately compensate for the relative complexity of case-mix, and therefore of cost, of inpatient cross-boundary flows. It is to be hoped that in future, records of cross-boundary flows of A & E, day and outpatients will become part of routine hospital information systems. However, it is regrettable that this information does not form part of the minimum data sets in the Korner recommendations on NHS information systems, currently being implemented by DHSS (NHS/DHSS Steering Group on Health Services Information, 1984a). The lead may have to come from Regions, since the absence of data on these flows is essentially a problem of sub-Regional resource allocation. At this level, the scale of the possible financial implications for Districts should be sufficiently large for Regions to contemplate the cost of mounting regular surveys.

COSTING CROSS-BOUNDARY FLOWS

RAWP Methods

RAWP methods for estimating the size of cross-boundary flows (and by implication, catchment populations) for resource allocation have been criticised not only on the grounds that day and outpatients are omitted and that the Net Flow method entials inappropriate assumptions about future changes in the extent of cross-boundary flows under a process of redistribution, but also that the cost allowance for cross-boundary flows may not be adequate. Under RAWP, cross-boundary flows by specialty were to be credited to the Region or Area providing treatment for patients from another Region or Area and debited from the Region or Area sending patients, at the national average specialty cost for the specialty of service provided (DHSS, 1976c, p.22, para. 2.17). These adjustments to targets are usually made two years in arrears of the flows taking place, but using current national average costs. Of course, these national average costs are not "current" in a real sense, since they are derived from a costing model which was developed using earlier data and simply revalued for inflation. They are expressed in terms of notional populations rather than sums of money, although in sub-Regional variants of RAWP, flows tend to remain as sums of money.

Criticisms of RAWP Methods

Criticisms of RAWP methods for dealing with the cost of flows exist on a number of levels. There are three criticisms of the manner in which credit for cross-boundary flows is given in RAWP: firstly, that RAWP compensation lags approximately two years behind the flows taking place; secondly, that credit is given in national RAWP (though usually not in contemporary sub-Regional RAWP) in the form of a population adjustment rather than in money terms; and thirdly, that the adjustment effects the RAWP target but not necessarily the current allocation of an authority. It seems that it would be feasible and relatively uncontroversial to answer the first two technical criticisms by using more up-to-date volume data in cross-boundary flow adjustments, and by making these adjustments in money terms (Smith, 1986). However, the third criticism which is often heard in the NHS, is not simply technical, but has a bearing on the basic objectives of RAWP. The RAWP process was designed to produce long-term resource targets. Authorities' allocations were to be moved progressively towards these targets. RAWP was not a method for determining current allocations. Thus, it is unfair and misguided to criticise RAWP for making cross-boundary flow adjustments to targets, but not to allocations.

However, the bulk of critics' attention has been focused not on the manner of cost compensation for flows, but on the level of the cost assumptions made. By using national average specialty costs for cross-boundary flows, RAWP was assuming that cases which cross boundaries receive care costing on average the same as those which do not. Critics have tended to argue that, in principle, more complex cases might be expected to cross boundaries and that RAWP compensation is therefore likely to be inadequate for inflows (Royal Commission on the National Health Service, 1978b). This immediately raised fears that the use of national average costs would create perverse incentives and distortions in access to care, with hospitals calculating the relative profitability or loss-making potential of importing or exporting particular sorts of cases, depending on local transfer prices (Radical Statistics Health Group, 1977, p.11). It was argued that this could have a detrimental effect on GPs' and patients' freedom of referral.

Criticism of the adequacy of the cost weighting for flows came particularly from

London. It was claimed that due to their special role in the National Health Service, the case costs of London hospitals might be above the national average with the tendency for more difficult and therefore, more costly cases to be sent to specialised centres in London. Thus, calls were made for more accurate estimates of the true costs to be used in RAWP; or at least the Thames Regional average costs for cases flowing into the Thames Regions (Thompson and Lally, 1980, p.48).

Since 1976, the likelihood of such problems of unfairness arising has been reduced by the gradual designation of certain specialised services attracting extensive inflows to main centres, as Regional specialties. Funds for these services are usually made available outside the RAWP process by "top-slicing" from overall Regional allocations and their flows are costed separately following the recommendations for supra-Regional specialties of the Advisory Group on Resource Allocation (DHSS, 1980b). Although the protection of a high proportion of the costs of Regional and supra-Regional Specialties may be seen as a logical response to RAWP's use of national average costs for cross-boundary flows, it has had implications for RAWP's pursuit of an equitable distribution of health care services. The amount spent on these categories of specialised services affects the size of the sum which remains available for redistribution. Since RAWP, the number of services eligible for special funding status has widened as part of a pragmatic response to the difficult problem of how to fund the activities of specialist centres, mainly teaching hospitals, in a system based on equitable finance by capitation. Thus, the emphasis has tended to be on the adequate protection of the costs of these specialised services with far less attention given to their equitable use. Local populations tend to make greater use of these services than the remainder of their notional catchments because of greater accessibility. The result of these developments is that an important part of NHS hospital expenditure is exempted from RAWP's criteria of equity. In principle, there seems no reason why steps should not be taken to ensure that Regional and supra-Regional services are used fairly by the whole of the populations they are supposed to serve.

Despite the development of Regional and supra-Regional specialties, the debate over costing of flows has continued, since it can still be argued that more complex cases will tend to be attracted into London and other main centres, not just in highly specialised fields, but also in the bread-and-butter, District specialties.

To criticise RAWP for making too crude an allowance for the costs of different sorts of cases crossing administrative boundaries, raises the relatively neglected policy issue of whether or not, given the scarcity of resources for health care, the treatment of more complex (and therefore, more expensive) cases should be fully compensated for in the funding process and therefore, effectively given priority over other, less complex cases. It may be that the health gains to be made from more straightforward cases are the same or greater than from complex cases, but at lower cost. From a societal point of view, health benefits might be maximised by a policy of restraining the numbers and proportion of complex cases in relation to simple cases. One way to effect this would be to refuse to provide full compensation for more complex cases. A related issue arises as to whether, even if the current case-mix is to be maintained, complex cases should be treated in places like central London where costs are known to be higher than elsewhere because of factors such as London weighting, higher wage costs in the London labour market, higher land prices, etc.. It might well be more economical (as well as more equitable) for the NHS to encourage the provision of more health care outside London. This would involve taking decisions about which flows should be encouraged and which not, rather than trying to cost the existing pattern of flows in minute detail. Decisions would also have to be made about the number of medical students to be trained in the capital and the number of beds in teaching hospitals required to support medical education.

With these caveats in mind, the criticisms of the RAWP approach to costing cross-boundary flows can be considered in two ways: firstly, what is the evidence that the use of national average specialty costs under-compensates the Districts providing treatment; and secondly, do differences between national average and actual costs affect RAWP targets appreciably?

The Evidence About the Cost of Flows and Its Significance for Targets

There is relatively little systematic evidence either to support or refute the claim that cross-boundary flows are more complex in case-mix than cases of residents because they are mainly to specialised services not available in the District of origin. However, the evidence which is available tends to throw doubt on this assertion. The majority of flows in District specialties seem to exist for reasons of convenience.

The Joint Working Group of representatives from DHSS and the Thames Regions on RAWP in London was critical of RAWP's use of national average specialty costs and sought to find a method of compensation which would be more sensitive to the "real costs" of services provided to non-residents. Regional and supra-Regional specialties could be excluded since their costs were largely safeguarded from the RAWP process through "top-slicing". In the event, the Joint Working Group was not able to recommend substantive changes to Thames sub-Regional RAWP methods because there were no data available on case complexity to substantiate the criticism of RAWP (DHSS and the Thames Regional Health Authorities, 1979, pp.38-40, paras. 6.1-6.9). The Advisory Group on Resource Allocation (AGRA) was the next official body to consider the issue of the use of national average specialty cost compensation for cross-boundary flows - this time in the context of national RAWP rather than RAWP in the Thames Regions. AGRA concluded that when the DHSS method of analysis of specialty costs by regression had been refined and the cost data provided in more detail, by changing from 12 specialty groups to 33 specialty groups, DHSS specialty costs worked reasonably well for cross-boundary flows of ordinary inpatient services. AGRA had commissioned a study comparing specialty cost estimates derived from the DHSS cost model with the actual costs of single specialty hospitals. The results were reassuring (DHSS, 1980b, p.19).

In one of the few studies to attempt to examine the case-mix of flows, Akehurst and Johnson (1980) were asked to find a method of adjusting sub-Regional RAWP targets for atypical, more expensive cross-boundary flows between Districts in the North Western Region. A number of Districts had argued that the costs of their imports to "centres of excellence" were insufficiently recognised in sub-Regional RAWP. The task was to discover if there was indeed any systematic tendency for more difficult cross-boundary cases to be treated in some AHAs rather than others, or whether a more costly than average case-mix in one specialty was offset by a less costly case-mix in another. In common with all researchers in this field, Akehurst and Johnson (1980) faced the problem of finding a good measure of case 'difficulty' which would be available for all the authorities in the Region and which could be easily converted into money terms. Length of inpatient stay was chosen as a proxy for 'difficulty' on the grounds that in general, intensity (costliness) and type of treatment had been found to be positively correlated with length of stay in the DHSS regression model used for estimating national average specialty costs for use in national RAWP. (This seems an odd justification for using legth of stay as a proxy for 'difficulty', since DHSS specialty costs are themselves estimated from the product of length of stay and hotel costs. The argument is, therefore, a circular one). Actual lengths of stay had to be adjusted to ovecome any confounding effects created by differences in efficiency between hospitals. 'Expected' lengths of stay were calculated based on knowledge of the Regional relationship between age, sex, diagnosis and length of stay for all cases. The 'expected' length of stay for each specialty, 1974-78 was compared with the Regional average length of stay for each specialty and the difference multiplied by the number of imported patients, giving an estimate of how many extra or fewer days of care would have to be provided by a health authority for imports, if it were of average efficiency. These days were then summed across all the health authorities in the Region. The sum was negative for four of the five years 1974 to 1978, implying that imported patients were on average slightly "easier" than residents in terms of their 'expected' lengths of stay. The extra or fewer patient days were then multiplied by per diem hotel costs, to show that for four out of the five years studied there would have been a net loss to health authorities if cross-boundary flows had been adjusted for case-mix using their method!

Akehurst and Johnson (1980) concluded that the overall effect of the lack of compensation for case-mix differences below the level of specialties in cross-boundary flows in most Districts was one of 'swings and roundabouts'. They could find no evidence in the North Western Region at least, of a major importing AHA or District being penalised by conventional RAWP methods. Most of the major importers appeared to be slight gainers from the existing system. The authors recognised that their use of length of stay as a proxy for 'difficulty' of cases was crude, but other evidence and subsequent developments have lent support to their conclusion that the degree of inequity involved in RAWP methods is small, if at all, in this respect.

Brazier (1986) points out that since inflows tend to be greatest in the relatively well-provided Districts in inner cities, where the most convincing explanation for their existence is on the grounds of convenience, it is unlikely that these cross-boundary flows will be significantly different in case-mix and therefore, cost, from cases generated within each District. Indeed, it may be argued that in the routine District specialties subject to RAWP, GPs outside the metropolitan centres are likely to refer more straightforward cases which they expect to have a shorter than average length of stay across administrative boundaries, rather than more difficult cases, where this involves patients going some distance. This would be to minimise inconvenience to the patient and his or her relatives, as well as to be better able to monitor the progress of patients. Furthermore, with the development of Regional and supra-Regional specialties benefiting from various degrees of protection from RAWP, it is increasingly likely since Akehurst and Johnson (1980) wrote, that the more complex and severe cases will be going to these specialties rather than the ordinary District specialties. Regional (or Multi-District Specialties as they are sometimes known) are usually funded nearer to their actual cost than to national average specialty costs. Seen in this way, the level of cost allowance for cross-boundary flows is a relatively minor deficiency in RAWP compared with the fact that day and outpatient flows are not recognised for compensation at all.

Brazier's (1986) discussion of the relative complexity of flows seems particulary applicable to a situation in which the majority of cross-boundary flows are between adjacent Districts in cities. However, recent research in progress in Birmingham tends towards rather different provisional conclusions. The study compares the relative complexity (as measured by length of stay) of cases from the Districts within the city of Birmingham treated at the Region's principal teaching hospital, the Queen Elizabeth Medical Centre, with cases from Districts outside Birmingham. The average length of stay for general surgery (an ordinary District specialty) was significantly higher in the patients from outside Birmingham than Birmingham patients at the hospital, indicating the possibility that the teaching hospital was receiving more difficult than average cases (Cooper, 1986). In the designated Regional specialties there was only a very slight (statistically non-significant) difference in average length of stay between Birmingham and outside Birmingham. By comparing cases at the same hospital, Cooper (1986) is able to overcome any confounding effects of relative efficiency of different hospitals. On the other hand, further research is needed to say with any confidence that the teaching hospital is treating more difficult cases. The possibility remains that the differences in length of stay observed are due to a distance effect which would be experienced by all hospitals. To test this hypothesis, Cooper (1986) has proposed to carry out the same comparison between distant and local cases in a non-teaching hospital in the West Midlands Region. In addition, there may be differences in the demographic characteristics of the two groups of patients affecting their relative lengths of stay, but not necessarily related to case complexity (eg. age and sex differences). Furthermore, length of stay is no more than a crude proxy for case complexity and says nothing directly about the resources consumed by the two groups of patients.

Although Cooper's study (Cooper, 1986) would tend to go against the conclusions of Akehurst and Johnson (1980), there are a number of important differences between the two studies which may help explain the findings. Firstly, Cooper (1986) looked at all cases treated at a single "centre of excellence" (ie.inflows and residents) and compared the length of stay of cases from Birmingham Districts and cases from outside Birmingham. Thus the comparison was not between cross-boundary flows and non-cross-boundary flows as in Akehurst and Johnson (1980), but between local and more distant cases. It is possible that a comparison of all cases crossing NHS boundaries with cases of District residents would reveal no significant difference in length of stay at the Queen Elizabeth Medical Centre, since the cross-boundary group would then include many more flows of convenience within Birmingham. Secondly, Cooper's study says nothing about outflows from the District in which the Queen Elizabeth Medical Centre operates nor about other Districts in the Region nor about specialties other than general surgery. Thirdly, Akehurst and Johnson (1980) looked at flows for each main specialty between all the Districts of the North Western Region and were thus in a position to observe a 'swings and roundabouts' effect, in which underfunding of one speialty of flows was compensated for by overfunding of another. It is theoretically possible that this occurs for Central Birmingham District where the Queen Elizabeth is situated. From a RAWP perspective the important question to answer for a District or Region with extensive flows is not so much, do RAWP methods accurately reflect the costs of inflows and outflows; but rather, what is the net effect of RAWP deductions and compensations for flows on the target?

Akehurst and Johnson (1980) in their study of the case-mix of inter-AHA and District flows showed that inpatient flows were, if anything, less complex (as measured by length of stay) than resident cases and that importing authorities were actually making a profit out of RAWP methods. They also worked out the size of the adjustment to allocations which would have been produced by using their more refined method of costing flows and found that the adjustments would have been very small. In only one AHA would the adjustment have exceeded 1% of the current allocation. In the same vein, West, Palmer, Patrick and Dodd (1980) carried out sensitivity analyses of the effects on Regional targets for NPIP services of doubling and then quadrupling the average cost of each specialty cost in the RAWP cross-boundary flow calculation. A factor of 2 produced very little change (less than 1% on average). A factor of 4 produced larger changes, with certain Regions consistently gaining and others losing. However, the changes only reached 3% to 4% of allocations in two out of fourteen Regions. In whichever way the DHSS specialty cost estimates were tested for robustness, the results differed by far less than the amount required to produce appreciable changes in RAWP targets. West et al (1980) concluded that the national average specialty costs used in national RAWP would have to be a grossly inaccurate proxy for the costs of treating cases for there to be any systematic over or under-provision for flows at Regional level. More especially, RAWP did not appear to be discriminating unfairly against high cost areas by its use of average costs derived from econometric estiamtes.

Although criticisms of the cost allowances for cross-boundary flows thus appear to be of little practical significance at Regional level, with Regional targets robust to changes in estimates of specialty costs, this begs the question of what happens sub-Regionally. Samples of cases are smaller, flow adjustments form a more significant element in RAWP targets and consistent patterns of import and export of patients exist between authorities. Yet Akehurst and Johnson (1980) concluded that any effects were self-cancelling within North Western RHA. There appear to be few, if any, other published studies of this issue.

The message from the evidence about the adequacy of the RAWP adjustments for cross-boundary flows would seem to be that at Regional level, and probably at District level as well, in most cases, criticisms of the level of the adjustment are of little practical significance for NPIP targets and allocations. Indeed national average costs by specialty continue to be used in national RAWP. For example, 1981/82 DHSS national average specialty costs were used in the calculation of 1985/86 Regional RAWP targets (DHSS, 1985b). However, there have been changes in the costing of psychiatric and mental handicap cross-boundary flows.

Costing Psychiatric and Mental Handicap Cross-Boundary Flows

RAWP used the national average specialty costs for psychiatry and mental handicap for compensation for flows of psychiatric and mental handicap patients at Regional level, in the same way as for NPIP services. A single case cost was thus calculated for the two specialties by dividing total expenditure by the total number of cases. However, because of the unusual length of stay distribution of psychiatric patients, the use of a single specialty cost has come under criticism. It has been argued that the use of a single case cost over-compensates Regions for in-flows of short-stay patients from other Regions, while under-compensating them for the cost of caring for long-stay patients. DHSS therefore, proposed to calculate separate case costs for patients in different length of stay groupings to provide a more equitable population adjustment for flows between Regions (DHSS, 1984a). The adjustment for old long-stay patients was not affected. The proposed changes were accepted by Regional Treasurers and first implemented in the 1985/86 national RAWP target calculations.

Cross-Charging Versus Costing Flows As A Means of Handling Flows

Criticism of the RAWP approach to costing cross-boundary flows has focused on the crudeness of the compensation using national average costs. Improvements have tended to be seen in terms of more detailed and sophisticated approaches to case costing. These solutions with their concern for better compensation for in-flows have much in common with recent proposals to introduce cross-charging into the NHS as a quasi-market solution to the problem of accommodating cross-boundary flows in a system of geographical redistribution (Brazier, 1986). Although cross-charging can take a variety of precise forms and can coexist to varying degrees with conventional NHS approaches to allocating resources, its essence consists of a situation in which one health authority negotiates a contract with another for its residents to receive specified services, at agreed costs and volumes, at the hospital of the other authority. Thus, the theory is that all flows will be properly costed. The proponents of cross-charging see numerous benefits flowing from its introduction to the NHS, particularly incentives for health authorities to seek out good quality, cost-effective suppliers of services for their residents and to provide good quality, cost-effective services themselves to attract patients from other Districts and hence revenue and jobs (Brazier, 1986). Cross-charging is also seen as a sensible way of making fairer use of the existing distribution of services. As was shown earlier in this chapter, a number of writers have considered that increasing patient mobility and accessibility is a better way of achieving equal access than relying on the physical redistribution of services from one geographical area to another (Dudley, 1977; Klein, 1977). Thus, Districts should not expect to provide all (nor necessarily the majority) of the services which they would like, in order to equalise their residents' consumption of services, but would arrange to "buy" services from Districts with "excess" or available capacity. To fund these purchases Districts could, for example, be given the residential component of their current RAWP target.

Specifically in the context of a discussion of RAWP cost weights for patient flows, cross-charging is perceived to have three advantages over the present system for the District supplying the service: firstly, under cross-charging, credit is received for in-flows in the year in which the services are provided, rather than by relying on adjustments to targets which are usually two years out-of-date; secondly, cross-charging provides an automatic adjustment to the District's income, whereas under RAWP an adjustment to a target for cross-boundary flows may not result in any increase in the actual allocation of the District providing the care for several years; and thirdly, cases treated from other Districts should be costed more accurately than under RAWP, with its use of relatively crude national average specialty costs. While the first two advantages are certain to be realised under cross-charging, the third is in some doubt. As the literature in this section has shown, under RAWP the accuracy of costing of cross-boundary flows is not an issue of prime importance, despite the fact that NHS managers have worried greatly about the use of national average specialty costs. However, under a proposed system of cross-charging in which Districts are required to search for the best suppliers and compete for patients from other Districts on the basis of cost and quality, detailed and accurate cost data will become vitally important. This presents problems, since at present, none of the available patient classification systems is likely to be adequate as a basis for comparing the relative efficiency of hospitals and setting charges in advance as part of a tendering process for cross-charging. Specialties are too heterogeneous to be used for setting prospective charges. Patient-based costing, even if it were feasible, could not be adopted, since it would amount to full-cost reimbursement and there would be no competitive incentives to improved efficiency built into the system. Diagnosis-Related Groups (DRGs) have been suggested as a means of classifying inpatients into relatively homogeneous cost groupings for cross-charging. But American research indicates that considerable variation in resource use may exist within DRGs (Horn, Starkey and Bertram, 1983). Their homogeneity may have been exaggerated. Expanding the number of groups to reduce DRG cost variation risks producing groups with too few cases to yield stable results (Sanderson, Craig, Winyard and Bevan, 1986). Even if DRGs were usable for inpatients, a further costing problem for cross-charging lies in the fact that there is no well-developed patient classification system for day and outpatient cases and no routine activity data is currently collected on these services in the NHS (Brazier, 1986). A system of Ambulatory Visit Groups (AVGs) similar to DRGs is under development, but it is too soon to be able to assess its relevance to the NHS (Fetter, Averill, Lichtenstein and Freeman, undated).

Costing is not the only issue which will have to be tackled before the advantages of cross-charging can be realised. Under cross-charging schemes, each District would be in direct control of its residents' use of services, thus eliminating the need to estimate the size of flows by complex methods of calculating catchment populations. Accordingly, a District would not be paid to treat a non-resident unless there was an explicit agreement to do so with the non-resident's District of origin. This raises the question of how emergencies, which comprise a large proportion of hospital work, should be dealt with. Enthoven (1985a) envisaged emergency cases being excluded from cross-charging arrangements and reimbursed at a standard cost. But is the definition of an "emergency" straightforward and how should such cases be reimbursed? There appears to be a conflict between being able to control the flow of residents across boundaries of a District and ensuring treatment for emergencies wherever they happen.

Cross-charging brings with it other difficulties, perhaps not immediately apparent. To be effective it requires that restrictions be placed on the traditional freedom of GPs and hospital consultants in the NHS to refer and admit patients wherever they choose in the Service, without reference to District management. Restrictions could be enforced if hospitals were only permitted to be reimbursed for patients from Districts with which they had service contracts. GPs would be effectively limited to referring patients to certain hospitals where they would be accepted as part of inter-District contracts. However, the medical profession would naturally resist such a development as an unacceptable violation of clinical freedom and against the best interests of patients.

Cross-charging lays bare other thorny issues. For example, under the current system most of the unpleasant rationing decisions about life-saving treatments fall to doctors where they often remain hidden from public view. Under cross-charging, District management would have to decide in advance, each year, how much to spend on different types of treatment for residents. If resident demand exceeded supply, District management and not clinicians would ultimately have to decide whether or not to deny treatment wherever the patient presented. The consequence could very well be a system highly susceptible to public pressure for life-saving treatment to be available in all circumstances, regardless of the overall balance of local health services and their contribution to the health status of the population (Bevan, 1986).

Cross-charging may present too many practical difficulties and undesirable consequences for widespread adoption in the NHS. However, it may have a more limited and specific role in helping secure equitable access to the highly specialised multi-District and Regional specialties which have developed since 1976 outside the RAWP process. These are currently concentrated in the teaching Districts and often, though not always, funded by "top-slicing". Thus, to varying degrees their costs are protected at "centres of excellence" where they are supposed to be available to all the residents of the Region or of a number of Districts in the case of multi-District specialties (MDS). Unsurprisingly, evidence suggests that patients living near the teaching hospitals make disproportionate use of these services. This is inequitable in RAWP terms since the funds for MDS and Regional specialties are unavailable for redistribution in relation to population needs. The NHS Regional Chairmen's Group is interested in using a system of cross-charging to fund Regional specialties and MDS to overcome this deficiency (South East Thames Regional Health Authority, 1986b). In South East Thames, the tentative proposal is to distribute the funds, normally "top-sliced", to the Districts which are nominally users of the Regional and multi-District specialties, on the basis of their populations. Districts would then be free to decide where and at what price, they would be prepared to buy these specialised services. In theory, this reform would ensure that each District, however peripheral, would have access to its "quota" of, for example, kidney transplants, each year, based on the annual incidence of kidney failure in the District population. Renal centres would have to compete for patients by offering good quality, economical treatment. It is theoretically possible that provincial Districts with lower input costs than metropolitan "centres of excellence" would find it financially (and perhaps politically also) preferable to provide certain specialised services themselves, which have hitherto been the preserve of established centres. For Regional specialties, cross-charging represents a rapid means of redistribution since user Districts would be given their share of the resources going into Regional specialties.

However, cross-charging for Regional specialties, shares many of the same drawbacks as cross-charging for ordinary District services (see above this section).

ESTIMATING CATCHMENT POPULATIONS AND COSTING FLOWS: IMPLICATIONS FOR POLICY

The foregoing discussion has tried to draw out the wider policy implications stemming from RAWP's treatment of cross-boundary flows. However, much of the literature and debate in the NHS on cross-boundary flows has tended to be narrowly technical. For example, concern has tended to focus on the adequacy of using DHSS national average costs as a measure of the cost of treating NPIP flows, on the grounds that flows are likely to be more complex than average. In fact, more accurate costing of inpatient flows is unlikely to alter Regional RAWP targets appreciably. Sub-Regionally, the situation is less clear-cut but it would seem sensible to follow Brazier's suggestion and to examine the robustness of targets at this level to changes in cost assumptions, before deciding whether or not to invest in the development of detailed costing procedures for inpatient flows (Brazier, 1986).

The absence of any compensation for day, outpatient and accident and emergency cross-boundary flows is likely to be far more important for Regional and District targets, as well as providing a disincentive to cost-effective day and outpatient care. Both national and sub-Regional RAWP should include an allowance for these flows. Routine data collection systems will have to be set up.

In the light of recent research, it seems that the issue of the costing of flows has received disproportionate attention as a potential source of unfairness. Though the costing of inpatient flows may not be perfect it would appear to be adequate. The main problem lies not so much for the District receiving extra in-flow cases, but for the District of residence of the patients who flow out across administrative boundaries and hinges on the lack of control of the District over outflows (Bevan and Brazier, 1985a). The existence of sizeable out-flows, common in many cities, poses grave difficulties to a District whose residents are consuming resources at an above average level in its task of trying to meet its RAWP target. Redrawing health authority boundaries to minimise the extent of flows and using more sophisticated formulae for estimating catchment populations (see Chapter Three), have both been proposed as possible remedies to this problem. It has been shown that neither proposal addresses the key issue, which is how Districts should control the supply of services to their residents and particularly, how they should control cross-boundary flows, to secure an equitable distribution and funding of services (Beech, Craig and Bevan, 1987). Under RAWP-type methods, an individual DHA with substantial flows can do little autonomously to promote an equitable consumption of services by its residents since its financial position is highly dependent on decisions to change provision and admit patients taken in the surrounding Districts. To promote equity in these circumstances requires the development of a means for health authorities to influence the behaviour of clinicians, either directly or indirectly. Regions are gradually becoming aware of this issue which RAWP chose to sidestep. Cross-charging represents a direct approach to influencing clinicians' behaviour by controlling access to resources through the establishment of formal agreements between provider and recipient Districts for packages of health care. By contrast, a number of Regions favour a more indirect, planning-based method in which clinicians' activities are shaped by relocating resources and services equitably through the funding of a Regional strategy (for example, North West Thames RHA, 1984a). Regional strategic management (RSM) as it has become known, is a planning-based approach to resource allocation which treats flows as amenable to changes which can be predicted. Under RSM, the effect on referral and flow patterns of future changes in the location of the supply of resources is simulated using techniques of gravity modelling. Clinical autonomy is not directly disturbed; rather, it is assumed that referral patterns will respond to changes in the spatial distribution of facilities (beds, manpower and revenue) (Bevan, 1986). The approach is discussed more fully in the next two chapters.

Cross-charging is an alternative "quasi-market" approach to the problem of flows in RAWP. In contrast to RSM, cross-charging involves direct interference by Districts in clinicians' freedom to refer or treat patients wherever they wish and amounts to a radical departure from the compromise between the independence of the medical profession and the authority of the state, on which the NHS is built. Under cross-charging, District managers rather than clinicians would ultimately have to take rationing decisions about who can be treated within the available finance, both for patients flowing in from other Districts and their residents in hospitals elsewhere (Brazier, 1986). It remains to be seen how politically acceptable this would be. Other problems are likely to arise with cross-charging. For example, although cross-charging promises to provide, among other benefits, a competitive environment with concomitant incentives to quality and efficiency, competition would have to exclude emergency treatment and chronic, long-term care and would be limited both by the number of producers which are effectively in competition in an area and by the willingness of DHAs to forego the opportunity of providing services themselves. Other hurdles include the difficulty of measuring cost and quality of services provided elsewhere.

In equity terms within a Region, cross-charging offers the potential benefit of enabling "deprived" Districts the opportunity of gaining immediate, direct access to services available in the better provided Districts without the painful necessity of physically redistributing resources. Although in the long term, "deprived" parts of the country are likely to want to provide their own health services locally, cross-charging may have a limited interim role for RAWP-gaining Districts, in securing access to services (particularly capital-intensive services) while they are being built up and before they are operational in such Districts. Specifically, the idea of using cross-charging is currently being floated as a permanent means of allocating MDS (or Regional specialties) fairly between District users (South East Thames Regional Health Authority, 1986b). However, there may be more conventional, managerial means of securing fairer access to and utilisation of, these services; for instance, by setting up out patient clinics in peripheral Districts, subsidising patient travel, or ensuring that peripheral GPs are given good information on treatments and their availability.

As Brazier (1986) points out, the various suggestions for ways of alleviating the problems encountered in dealing with cross-boundary flows under a policy of achieving equity, are not mutually exclusive. Cross-charging could be used in a limited way for particular services (eg. hip replacement) in conjunction with a redrawing of the most idiosyncratic boundaries to reduce the scale of flows for acute services (eg. in London) and a policy of Regional strategic management of equity (eg. for major capital developments). Furthermore, each proposal for easing the tension between the existing pattern of flows and the long-term pursuit of geographical equity comes up against two underlying issues which are unlikely to be resolved easily; firstly, the extent to which extra money can be found for the NHS so that equity can be pursued in part by a process of "levelling up" involving the elimination of a large proportion of the flows caused by scarcity; and secondly, the extent to which the use of health services (and especially flows) can be "planned" or influenced by health authorities in a system which supports a high degree of clinical freedom. The resolution of both issues is ultimately a political rather than a technical exercise.

CHAPTER SEVEN

RAWP AND PLANNING

INTRODUCTION

While a great deal of effort has gone into technical criticisms of the RAWP formula, fewer writers have grappled with how resource allocation and planning can and should be related. This is one of the most important strategic issues and is the subject of this chapter. In the early years, the two processes were inadequately integrated in the NHS. An American commentator in a comparative study of health care systems saw this as one of the principal issues remaining to be resolved by the NHS:

'Health planning as reorganization succeeded in creating a new administrative structure and in institutionalizing a formal planning process. Health planning as resource allocation succeeded in making the central government explicitly recognise trade-offs among alternative resource configurations within the health sector. Neither kind of planning, however, has succeeded in achieving policy integration and implementation. Regional disparities in the provision of health care services remain, whether measured in terms of expenditures, hospital beds, or manpower. The priorities outlined in the Priorities Document and in The Way Forward remain unmet. And the NHS remains a health service characterized by hospital-centred care.'
(Rodwin, 1984, p.177)

Bevan, Copeman, Perrin and Rosser (1980, p.156) made a similar point:

'The problem facing authorities is that, while the RAWP principles have overcome the inertia of maintaining the status quo, they provide no basis for a different system. This is because decisions about resource allocation cannot be sensibly separated from decisions about deployment.'

One of the principal themes of this book is that RAWP methods are reliable guides for deciding RHA allocations, are probably good indicators of the fairness of use of services by DHA populations, but fail to provide an adequate framework for devolving decisions to DHAs. Targets may fairly indicate how resources in total ought to move between DHA populations but it is not sensible to require DHAs to bring this about, particularly in cities where there are large cross-boundary flows between DHAs. The purpose of this chapter is to describe, by drawing on the literature, how RAWP methods were, for a time, seen as an appropriate means of devolving responsibilities for redistribution away from the levels where they could be most reasonably tackled. The focus of this is sub-Regional allocation and the tasks of RHAs, but the origins of the problem lie in the separation of resource allocation from planning within DHSS in the 1970s. This chapter begins with descriptions of their separate development.

THE SEPARATION OF RAWP FROM PLANNING SERVICE PRIORITIES IN DHSS IN THE 1970S

Changing Concepts of Planning and Resource Allocation

One of the principal objectives of the 1974 reorganisation was to get away from the "disjointed incrementalism" of the past which had resulted in the prolongation of pre-existing patterns of resource distribution (Gray and Hunter, 1983, p.419). Butts provides a helpful textual analysis of the various reorganisation documents produced by the Heath Government aimed at producing a comprehensive, rational planning system for the NHS (Butts, Irving and Whitt, 1981, pp.51-55). The 1972 Conservative White Paper (DHSS, 1972b) stated an intention to integrate the processes of planning and financial allocations:

'The allocation of available funds to health authorities will be designed progressively to reduce the disparities between the resources available to different Regions and to achieve standards and improvements in services with due regard to national, regional and area priorities.' (Para. 60)

'The allocation of funds by the regional authorities will be closely integrated with the planning process so that plans are based realistically on the level of funds likely to be made available.' (Para. 153)

'The estimates produced as part of the planning process will be the framework for a budgeting system designed both to give overall control and to provide functional budgets which will help individual managers to exercise detailed control over resources...' (Para. 159)

The reorganisation circular HC(73)3 (DHSS, 1973) stated:

'Accordingly, the main management control to be exercised by one level over another will be the preliminary allocation of resources and the setting of guidelines to the level below, followed by detailed review and approval of plans covering the whole range of services and monitoring of performance in relation to plans.'

This would appear to indicate an iterative process of setting financial guidelines, followed by approving plans, followed by making definitive financial allocations. The subsequent development of policies for resource allocation and care group priorities tends to indicate that the cycle never materialised. When the Resource Allocation Working Party was established in May 1975, its remit demonstrated that its task was seen as separate from the parallel activities which were taking place at the same time in the DHSS leading to the promulgation of the consultative document Priorities for Health and Personal Social Services (DHSS, 1976a). Soon after, the 1976-77 planning guidelines (DHSS, 1976b) published methods for establishing financial allocations based on criteria distinct from those used for general planning, thus confirming the separation of the two processes (Butts, Irving and Whitt, 1981, p.64). Butts' review of the first round of Regional Strategic Plans provides evidence that different criteria were indeed used by RHAs for calculating financial allocations as against establishing levels of provision of different services in Strategic Plans. He sees this as the product of 'muddled thinking' within DHSS and NHS (Butts et al, 1981, p.84), but this alone would seem an inadequate explanation. A fuller understanding of the relationship (or lack of it) between resource allocation and service planning emerges with a consideration of the organisation, functions and assumptions of the DHSS and how these factors both reflect and determine the character of the NHS.

Planning and Resource Allocation at DHSS Level

Irving argues that the failure to adopt an integrated approach to planning and resource allocation reflected in part at least the working of the DHSS in the mid-and late 1970s and its failure to provide an authoritative source of Strategic direction to the NHS after the RAWP report appeared (Butts et al, 1981, pp.42-5). As one of the largest and most complex Central Government Departments, DHSS boasted a series of different groups with different roles and perspectives involved wholly or in part in planning, developing and funding health services after RAWP. Among the participants were the Regional Liaison Divisions responsible for maintaining close contact with the NHS through the Regions, the various Policy Branches and the Service Development Group responsible for originating guidance on levels of provision and "good practice", the Finance Divisions responsible for the process of financial allocations and senior officials close to the Minister whose prime responsibility was to service the Secretary of State in discharging his Parliamentary duties.

Irving's account makes three crucial points about DHSS policies following the 1974 reorganisation. First, she argues that there was a lack of integration between the detailed policies and programme budgets which appeared in early sets of planning guidelines after the 1974 reorganisation and the first Regional Strategic Plans. The DHSS programme budget was intended to ensure that policy commitments and resource assumptions were reconciled but this did not occur. She accounts for this in terms of the inadequacy of NHS financial information systems and the reluctance of Ministers and policy branches in the DHSS to accept financial constraints: policy branches tend to pursue the sectional interest of a particular care group, and the overall Services Development Group failed to arbitrate between these claims since it did 'not have to face the problems of running the NHS and reconciling competing claims on resources'. Formal, direction contact with the health authorities which had the responsibility of trying to provide a comprehensive service within a fixed budget was the task of officials in the Regional Liaison Divisions and not officials in the policy divisions. Officials in the policy divisions were in close contact not with NHS management but with various pressure groups and with the professional advisory committees of doctors, nurses, midwives, etc., who ensured that they were made fully aware of the deficiencies in the services for particular client groups. As a result, Irving claims, health authorities were frustrated by the remoteness of care group policy makers from the new problem of planning to a fixed budget and the preoccupation of the most senior officials with political policy making in the service of their Ministers rather than with achieving results in the NHS. In common with other parts of the public sector, the mid 1970's was a period of painful adjustment to the need to reconcile the desirability of implementing programmes with their likely cost. The decision ten years later, on the recommendation of the Griffiths Enquiry (DHSS, 1983) to set up an NHS Management Board at DHSS level can be seen as a response to the persistence of the problem in DHSS that there appeared to be no individual or group of people with specific responsibility for providing a clear strategic lead to the Service.
Second, she argues that the effect of the RAWP formula was 'conspicuously absent' from the central planning system:

'Although it might be argued that the main concern in developing national priorities is the distribution between client groups and that the distribution between geographical areas is an entirely separate issue, it is clear from practical experience in the NHS that the two approaches need to be reconciled.'
(Butts et al 1981, p.44)

Irving explains this in terms of the structure and working of the Department in the 1970s: the fact that the Services Development Group worked separately from the Regional Group; links between Service Development and Finance were tenuous through the Public Expenditure Survey Committee (PESC) and the programme budgeting exercises; and the whole was uncoordinated with RAWP. (There have been significant changes within the DHSS since Irving wrote. The potential of the new NHS Management Board to address itself to the sorts of issues raised in this section is discussed in the conclusions to this chapter.) It is possible that Irving overstates the lack of coordination within DHSS at this time. For example the Regional Liaison Divisions were in a position to see the inequalities in provision which existed between different parts of the country and to point these out to the Services Development Group.

Third, Irving questions the assumptions of DHSS about appropriate levels of devolution of responsibility to health authorities and the capacity of the new planning system to effect change. In financial terms, health authorities were given the freedom to manage as they judged best. National priorities were seen as broad guidance only, since the planning system would offer the main control mechanism to keep AHAs on course. Varley (1982) highlights how Ministers saw functional and geographical redistribution in a straightforward way as simultaneous and complementary policies with this quotation from the 1976 Priorities Document:

'The Resource Allocation Working Party... has recommended that allocations to regions should aim progressively to reduce disparities between them. ...Those regions which gain extra resources from this policy should be able to achieve an above average improvement of their services; those whose allocations are restricted will need to scrutinise all their services with particular care, especially the relatively expensive ones such as the specialist hospital services.'
(DHSS, 1976a, p.27, para.4.15)

Experience of health authorities since 1976 has shown how difficult it has been to implement these policies and the extent to which they have conflicted. Irving contends that Ministers and DHSS had naive expectations of the ability of health authorities to respond simultaneously to: the wide range of guidance being offered; the move from an incremental approach to service developments towards rational comprehensive planning requiring complex changes in health services; and the requirement to cut certain services in order to redeploy resources elsewhere as cash limits were introduced. She claims that:

'The Department was under the illusion that because it had designed a planning system and got the central part working, it could now assume that the whole system worked.'
(Butts et al, 1981, p.45)

It seems unlikely that experienced senior officials were as naive as Irving asserts but as Butts points out (Butts et al 1981, p.71),DHSS at that time had no real mechanism at its disposal for ensuring policy implementation and since DHSS and Treasury were reluctant to earmark more than a relatively small proportion of the NHS budget (e.g. joint finance) for particular priorities, it could not exert influence in the only way left open. Furthermore, pressure groups in opposition to the local implementation of national policy, have continued to embarrass Ministers and on occasions compelled them to withdraw tough, unpopular decisions which were nonetheless in line with RAWP and priorities.

Central-Local Relations in the Health Service

Mullen (1978, p.7) suggests that the lack of integration of the planning and resource allocation processes far from being the result of naivety may have been a means (however imperfect) to resolve conflicts between the two seemingly incompatible objectives of the NHS planning system of maximum delegation downwards coupled with overall central development control in recognition of the fact that the Health Service is centrally funded but with a marked degree of local autonomy. In this context, it can be seen as preferable to allocate monetary resources via an agreed central formula, but allow local health authorities extensive freedom to deploy these resources as they see fit in the light of local circumstances. In another sense, such an arrangement may be seen as implicitly recognising the importance of clinical autonomy at local level and its influence on policy implementation.

Indeed studies of central-local relations in the NHS in the 1970s and 1980s have shown the tendency of health authorities to frustrate and avoid the implementation of central government policies (Haywood and Alaszewski, 1980; Haywood and Elcock, 1980). Kenneth Lee reminds us that:

> 'Whilst it might be expected that local plans and expenditure be consistent with national economic and social policies, this tends to over-simplify the delicate nature of independence afforded to the subordinate agencies or periphery.'
> (Lee 1977, p.211)

As a result, DHSS priorities at that time, were not firm guides to action, but could be seen (and were often treated) as considerations to be borne in mind, which set the limits of policy and informed the content of negotiations between tiers (Haywood, 1983, p.427). In this context, any integration of planning and resource allocation would necessitate a change in central-local relations within the Health Service with the setting of more detailed objectives expressed in terms of finance, manpower and other resources, followed by monitoring of actual expenditure and services delivered to ensure that objectives had been met. In such a system, financial allocations might be put in jeopardy if policies were pursued which were inconsistent with DHSS guidelines (Royal Commission on the NHS, 1978a, p.26, para. B4.11). The seeds of such an approach can be seen in DHSS policy since 1982, with the introduction of various mechanisms of accountability for efficient use of resources, such as Performance Indicators and Regional Reviews. These measures were contrary to the then Secretary of State's (Patrick Jenkin) enthusiasm for devolution of responsibility for decisions in the Health Service to Districts and individual clinicians, but were largely forced on him by the House of Commons Public Accounts Committee which had been very critical of the absence of effective methods publicly to monitor the extent of the implementation of policy by health authorities and the efficiency with which they used public resources (House of Commons Public Accounts Committee, 1981 and 1982). However, in the mid 1970s civil servants had to find other ways of managing inherent tensions between levels and between objectives in the NHS.

RAWP's View

The RAWP Report (DHSS, 1976c, p.8, para. 1.5) stated:

> 'Resource allocation is concerned with the distribution of financial resources which are used for the provision of real resources. In this sense it is concerned with the means rather than the end. We have not regarded our remit as being concerned with how the resources are deployed. This must be a matter for the administering Authorities and is essentially

part of their policy-making functions in response to central guidelines on national policies and priorities.'

Whilst Irving's critique explains how RAWP became separated from the planning system, it does not fully explain why RAWP took this view of planning and resource allocation and followed its chosen approach. The first point to remember is that at the time when RAWP was sitting the various "priorities" documents had not yet been published. Thus there was no strategic planning framework for RAWP to relate its proposals to. However, RAWP's approach may further be understood given the way the policy problem of geographical inequalities in Health Service resources was conceived of at the time the Working Party was established. The principal concern of all those involved was to deal with financial inequalities at Regional level. The evidence of sub-Regional inequalities had only recently been revealed in 1975 and its implications for developing a fairer resource allocation mechanism had not been thought through. Thus much of RAWP's time and energies went into devising a formula-based approach suitable for use at RHA level. Since RHAs did not deliver health services themselves, the process of making financial allocations did not need to be integrated with the procedure for Regional planning.

Furthermore, by basing RHA allocations on RAWP targets, as Bevan et al (1980, p.147) point out, the separation of resource allocation from planning is useful for the DHSS 'because it means that regional plans cannot reasonably be bids for extra resources'. This point is developed below. The old bidding process was discredited in the eyes of the Working Party by its association with the pre-1970 incremental approach which had perpetuated inherited inequalities in resources. In pre-RAWP days the Regions submitted rival proposals for capital developments which were in effect, claims for additional resource and each year the Ministry of Health had the uneasy task of deciding between them. The RAWP procedure is particularly attractive in a period of stringency since it provides independent arbitration of conflicting claims for resources. 'Apparently this "taking allocations out of politics" appealed to the administrators who composed the bulk of RAWP's membership' (Pollitt, 1984, p.48). It is likely that it appealed also to Ministers. Some critics have implied that RAWP was an explicit rationing device introduced at a time of stringency to succeed normative planning (which implies some notion of a minimum acceptable level of services) as articulated through the 1962 Hospital Plan, which was becoming discredited. However, the timing of RAWP and the imposition of cash limits may have been coincidental since RAWP started its work before the public expenditure crises of the mid-1970s hit the welfare state.

It would be misleading to imply that RAWP was unaware that resource allocation and deployment interacted:

'Resource allocation will clearly have an important influence on the discharge of those functions [policy-making, planning and decision-making in relation to national policies and priorities] and be the most critical guideline within which they have to be discharged.'

'Whilst as we have said earlier, resource allocation is not directly concerned with the way in which resources are actually deployed, it has of course a very considerable influence on the planning process... The formulation of resource targets is clearly an important first step in planning the provision of services... we draw particular attention to the importance of following through our proposals effectively in the planning process which will make their impact explicit.'
(DHSS, 1976c, p.8, para. 1.5 and p.85, para. 6.34)

However, there were no recommendations as to how this should be recognised formally and at the time, RAWP was probably in no position to do so. RAWP appeared to have little information from, or contact with, the group responsible for drawing up the first DHSS Programme Budget and 1976 Priorities Document (DHSS, 1976a). Furthermore RAWP's remit was specifically to consider the method of allocation of financial resources. It could not have been expected to tackle all the planning and implementation problems which beset DHSS as well! In 1976 there was no methodology at DHSS level to reconcile competing policies. Programmes tended to be in conflict with one another and control over implementation of policy within the Health Service tended to be limited to exhortation with little effect. For example the 1976 Priorities Document showed that expenditure was contrary to declared policies. In this context and with very little time at its disposal, RAWP sensibly confined itself to its remit. The responsibility for integrating resource allocation with planning and improving implementation and accountability, lay outside RAWP.

Central Developments After RAWP

The lack of formal integration between RAWP and planning was rationalised by adopting the principle that RAWP was to guide the allocation of resources between competing health authorities, while planning priorities would guide allocations within health authorities (Bevan, et al, 1980, p.175). However, in reality things were less clear-cut and these two processes came into conflict.

In 1979, the Information Sub-Group of the Standing Group on NHS Planning, commenting on the fact that resource allocation and planning guidance as embodied in the DHSS Programme Budget were based on separate criteria and implemented separately, concluded that:

'any integration would be a complex operation which would not be embarked upon at the present time.'
(Quoted in Butts et al, 1981, p.177)

The complexity is not surprising given that RAWP and the Programme Budget (DHSS, 1976a; DHSS, 1977a) were developed independently to carry out different tasks and adopted different methodologies as a result of their objectives and the availability of suitable data. Thus the seven service categories used by the RAWP allocation method were chosen because they fitted existing DHSS accounting and cost categories, enabling precise financial targets to be calculated. The client groups used in the DHSS Programme Budget were defined so as to be appropriate for planning the development of services in line with Departmental priorities. The client groups could not easily be costed with available data and certainly not with the accuracy required for resource allocation, but since the Programme Budget was seen as a strategic planning tool and its priorities as merely illustrative, accurate costings were not regarded as necessary.

In 1978 the Procedures and Costing Sub-Group of the Standing Group on NHS Planning had studied the problems of integrating RAWP and the Programme Budget systems. The Group had concluded that merging the two systems would not only be very complex but also impracticable because of the different costing methods employed. It was impossible to cost services by care group with the accuracy required for resource allocation purposes. Furthermore, while a Programme Budget could be built up for each Region using the national method, taking into account Regional population size and structure, etc., the Programme Budget methodology included no specific allowance for differential population morbidity and the Group was against RAWP SMRs in this context since this would involve accepting a further set of assumptions and uncertainty:

'So far as relating Regional and national priorities is concerned, it is possible to develop indicators which relate expenditure by programmes to population weighted on RAWP principles. However, there are considerable uncertainties involved in estimating expenditure and population weights for

individual programmes on a comparable basis for each Region.'
(DHSS, 1978, para. 11)

The Sub-Group felt that it was desirable to develop a variety of indicators using different assumptions as an aid to judgement on plans but that they could not be used rigidly by DHSS to make financial allocations. Although Health Service costing systems have been improved since 1978, the question of reconciling the two systems does not appear to have been taken up again, perhaps because DHSS no longer publishes its Programme Budget for the future.

The Royal Commission on the NHS which reported the following year, was perplexed as to whether any attention was being given to DHSS priorities or not, in the way resources were allocated. The Members agreed with the verdict of the House of Commons Expenditure Committee that:

'the expenditure planning and priority setting of DHSS should be synchronised so as to enable Parliament to examine the relationship between the two.'
(Quoted in Royal Commission on the National Health Service, 1979, p.56, para. 6.17)

They went on:

'...even after listening to careful explanation by representatives of the DHSS about the way in which the needs of particular priority groups are taken into account in the allocation of resources... we remain mystified.'
(Royal Commission on the National Health Service, 1979, p.56, para. 6.17)

SERVICE PRIORITIES AND RESOURCE ALLOCATION IN THE NHS

This account of the early separation of RAWP from planning at the centre naturally leads on to questions about what this implied for health authorities. The literature on this aspect is concerned with two main points: one is the nature of RAWP targets and their implied incentive effects; and the other is the problem of trying to implement geographical and care group redistribution sub-Regionally in the NHS with little or no growth in resources.

The Incentive Effects of Target Composition

RAWP's decision not to consider the planning implications of resource allocation in any detail had a variety of consequences within the formula itself. One example of RAWP's failure to link service priorities to resource allocation was the way in which the seven service categories used in the RAWP formula (non-psychiatric inpatients, day patients and outpatients, community health services, ambulance services, mental illness inpatient services, mental handicap inpatient services and FCA administration) were combined according to weightings derived from their proportions of past expenditure. There was no discussion in the report of the question of whether the historical distribution was appropriate. The proportions used had the drawbacks that they were the product not of conscious decisions but of piecemeal modifications to services. The expenditure data on which they were based were already several years old when they came to be used in the formula, thus emphasising the historical nature of the exercise (Creese, Darby, Palmer and Patrick, 1978). The Black Report criticised the use of past expenditure proportions in the formula and recommended that the categories 'should reflect not current distribution of expenditure, but that which is aimed at in the planning of services' (DHSS, 1980a, p.264, para. 8.58). Creese et al (1978) used the programme budget set out in the DHSS consultative document on health and social services priorities (DHSS, 1976a) to derive the weights to be attached to the seven service categories used in the RAWP formula and then employed the new weights in the formula. The percentage changes in total Regional targets were marginal (ie. the formula was relatively robust - changes in assumptions did not alter the basic pattern of reallocation), but the changes were considerably larger expressed as a proportion of the sums actually redistributed by RAWP. Creese and colleagues concluded that agreed NHS priorities should explicitly influence the weights used in the formula as a preliminary step towards the proper integration of planning and resource allocation and stressed the basic, but often overlooked, fact that 'a reassessment of service priorities is likely to alter resource needs as calculated by RAWP'.

These criticisms of RAWP methods and their subsequent implementation are a valid comment on the uncoordinated way in which DHSS introduced RAWP and promulgated its first Programme Budget (DHSS, 1976a), but cannot apply to the Working Party itself. They overlook the fact that the 1976 Priorities Document was not in existence when RAWP was deliberating. Thus, there were no planned, future expenditure proportions available which RAWP could have included in the formula. No doubt this could have been changed over the years since RAWP was introduced, but in 1975/76 there was nothing RAWP could do except use historical data, unless a decision had been taken elsewhere in DHSS to link the RAWP exercise explicitly with the evolving work on the DHSS Programme Budget. RAWP was appointed to develop a method for allocating financial resources according to the needs of administrative populations, not to make policy judgements about the appropriate proportion of NHS expenditure which each care group should receive. The Working Party had limited time to accomplish its task and reasonably chose to restrict its deliberations to its remit.

Resource allocation through RAWP pointing in a different direction from service priorities is most clear for services for the mentally ill and handicapped. In brief, the approach when the RAWP formula was introduced was to estimate for each Region an expected number of inpatients based on national average rates of mental illness and mental handicap hospitalisation. It was assumed for resource allocation purposes, that for Regions with fewer than average numbers of inpatients other Regions were treating their patients and their targets were reduced accordingly, regardless of whether this was the case or not. While there are various technical objections to this methodology and queries as to the cost data used (Senn and Shaw, 1978), its principal disadvantage lay in the perverse incentives it held out to Regions which were being encouraged through DHSS priorities to develop community care of the mentally ill and mentally handicapped. If Regions followed a policy of community care they would be penalised since they would reduce their number of inpatients and would have a lower number than would be expected at the national average hospitalisation rate. This would mean for RAWP purposes that the mental illness component of their target would also be reduced, since it was assumed in the formula that these "missing" patients were being treated outside the Region in other hospitals (Bevan et al, 1980, p.148).

In making sub-Regional RAWP allocations all Regions have now abandoned the original method for calculating the mental illness and mental handicap element of RAWP targets. Regions use a variety of different funding approaches congruent with policies for the gradual run-down of large mental illness and mental handicap hospitals and their replacement with community-based facilities.

Redistribution Without Growth

In the late 1970s and the 1980s the NHS was faced with a variety of external constraints and pressures while at the same time it was given a set of demanding policy objectives by central government. A policy of geographical redistribution had to be implemented in the context of an ageing population making increasing demands on the Health Service, reduced growth in total health care resources, and a strategy of developing the care of hitherto-neglected patient groups and community-care alternatives to institutional provision. A further complicating factor was the existence of deprived Areas and Districts within RAWP-losing (so-called "well-off") Regions and the consequent need to ensure that such places received due recognition in sub-Regional RAWP. The separation of planning from resource allocation at DHSS level described earlier in this Chapter would have been far less significant had the NHS been experiencing a period of expansion while RAWP was being implemented. However, from the mid-1970s health spending in the UK grew very slowly in real terms compared with the late 1960s and early 1970s. The first major slowing down in the growth of expenditure coincided almost exactly with the publication of the RAWP report, by which time the Working Group had already agreed its methods based on the assumption that redistribution would occur primarily through allocating differential growth. Yet the annual growth rates which were set in the late 1970s allowed little room for manoeuvre for Authorities trying to build up their priority services. Increases in funding were frequently absorbed in inflation and demographic change so that certain Authorities experienced a cut in resources in real terms.

The RAWP Report recommended that its methods be applied to allocations below Regional level, with only minor amendments as required (DHSS, 1976c, pp.37-8). Chapter Four reviews criticisms that at sub-Regional level the stability of a number of the variables, particularly SMRs is open to question with possibly major fluctuations in targets as a result. In relation to planning sub-Regionally, a more important issue is the sensitivity of a formula-based approach to variations in local circumstances. RAWP went as far as stating that local factors of a practical nature must be taken into account in the interpretation of progress towards targets (DHSS, 1976c, p.45). For example, it was conceivable that a particular District would always be kept above its indicated target because of the impact on its services of social deprivation (DHSS, 1976c, p.41); but there is no discussion of the possibility that the determination of the targets themselves could be based on local circumstances and planning objectives. The Working Party placed a higher premium on ensuring that targets were established 'on a compatible basis' throughout the country to ensure, for example, that neighbouring Districts in different Regions did not use 'different and incompatible criteria'. Although the report does refer to the possible relationship between District resource allocation and local plans and priorities, the point is expressed opaquely and is not developed sufficiently to attract the reader's attention. The Report seems to indicate that resource allocation is a prior process (certainly a separate one) within the constraints of which, planning and resource deployment decisions have to take place:

'Differences will and should of course continue to exist between localities within as well as between RHAS, but these should only be as a result of planning decisions taken within the framework of compatible allocation systems.'
(DHSS, 1976c, p.38, para. 3.3.1)

While Regions have adhered to a greater or lesser extent to the methods in the RAWP report, the basic intention of RAWP that resource allocation should be through an objective formula largely separate from the planning system was fulfilled. However, the fact that different Regions do use different methods to calculate District targets, does affect the size of District targets. Descriptions of some of the modifications which have been made by Regions to the factors in the formula (e.g. population base chosen (Chapter Three), calculation of cross-boundary flows (Chapter Six), inclusion of social deprivation factors (Chapter Five), etc.) is given elsewhere in this literature review. In this section the focus is specifically on the impact of resource allocation methods on service development and redeployment of resources between care groups.

A number of writers have tried to characterise the way in which changes determined by RAWP have been implemented within Regions. Maynard and Ludbrook reviewing the first three years of RAWP identified 'cause for considerable concern about some aspects of the reaction to the RAWP changes' and concluded:

'It seems clear that inadequate notice is being taken of centrally defined priorities.'
(Maynard and Ludbrook, 1980a, p.305)

Bosanquet's assessment of the consequences of RAWP looked particularly at the conflicts which had not been recognised but which were becoming apparent after the first three years of RAWP, between the objectives of increasing the level of provision in the under-target RHAs (e.g. Trent), redistributing resources to under-target Areas within high spending Regions, improving services for priority care groups, particularly in Districts with teaching hospitals, and responding to social deprivation in the inner cities by improving basic community health eervices (Bosanquet, 1980). The conflicts appeared to be resulting in a slowing down of the pace of redistribution, particularly between inner and outer London. Similarly, Bevan et al (1980, p.148) gave an example of a Region in which above-target Areas had inadequate psychiatric services (a national priority), but to develop these services would have pushed the Areas' actual expenditure even further in excess of their targets.

The most serious weakness of RAWP from Bosanquet's point of view was that:

'...it put the fighting of inequalities in the acute services well in front of action against inequalities between client groups and between classes.'
(Bosanquet, 1980, p.215)

Although two case studies by Davidson (1980) and Richardson (1984) appear to provide support for this conclusion, closer examination shows that the money secured by acute services after 1976 was often the result of the necessity to fund the revenue consequences of recently-completed acute hospitals from within their own budgets, rather than a direct effect of RAWP itself. An important side effect of the introduction of RAWP was the ending of DHSS funding of these revenue consequences. Davidson (1980) and Richardson (1984) were based on two Area Health Authorities, one being a "RAWP-gainer" and the other a "RAWP-loser". Similar trends were identified by Jeffries (1978) who monitored the impact of resource allocation in the late 1970s in the Oxford Region and concluded that community hospitals and "social" beds for the elderly were being closed to protect acute services in the main centres.

The sorts of problems which financially constrained health authorities have faced in implementing RAWP below Regional level, in conjunction with policies on care group priorities (which the above examples hint at) were accurately foreseen by Klein as soon as the final RAWP Report was published in 1976 (Klein, 1976). He recognised that with low levels of NHS expenditure growth, meaningful redistribution could only be achieved by cutting or freezing the allocations to the over-target Regions. In addition, an even more marked cut-back in expenditure would be required in over-target AHAs within Regions because of the greater extent of resource inequality at sub-Regional level. Furthermore, he estimated that to achieve anything like the objectives set in the 1976 Priorities Document (DHSS, 1976a) in AHAs with frozen or reducing budgets, would require major cuts in acute services. This would entail highly visible closures and have major political costs. Klein proposed that for the policy to be realistic, extra monies should be specifically set aside at national level for allocation to AHAs thus affected, in order to reduce the frictional costs of introducing desirable changes in resource distribution.

Social Deprivation and Inner Cities

In Chapter Five the argument over social deprivation and how it should be allowed for in resource allocation to health authorities was reviewed. The conclusion was that the search for a social deprivation weighting to be incorporated in global targets was misguided. Instead the Chapter argued for an approach based on planning. In this Chapter it is apposite to discuss what is perhaps one of the most striking seeming contradictions in government policy between RAWP and the policies of the Inner Cities Directorate of the Department of the Environment (DOE). The attainment of RAWP targets will result in a major shift of resources away from inner London in contrast with the recognition by other government departments of London's special problems. While recognising the possible role of social deprivation in determining the level of need for health care, the RAWP Working Party refrained from including a weighting for social deprivation in the formula for two reasons: firstly because it was felt that data were not available to quantify the relationship between quality of housing environment, etc., and need for health services; and secondly, because the RAWP judged that dealing with social deprivation was the province of other social programmes and that it would be inappropriate for the NHS to try to compensate for poverty, bad housing etc. except in so far as they affected mortality rates (DHSS, 1976c, p.11, para. 1.16 and pp.14-15, para.2.5). While approving the latter statement as a long-term principle, Buxton and Klein raised the legitimate question of:

'...what actually happens if the provision of health care is reduced in otherwise deprived areas, without any administrative mechanism for ensuring that the "deficiences" of the other relevant services will actually be remedied.'
(Royal Commission on the National Health Service, 1978b, p.13)

The GLC Health Panel was more strongly critical of the omission of deprivation by RAWP and of the crudity of the deprivation weighting devised and recommended for use in calculating targets by the DHSS and Thames Regions' Joint Working Group on RAWP (DHSS and Thames Regional Health Authorities, 1979, pp.6-17). The Health Panel argued that a high level of social deprivation may result in an increased need for health care, over and above any resulting increase in morbidity (e.g. by lowering the threshold for admission and increasing length of stay) (GLC Health Panel, 1984, p.15). Inclusion of a deprivation factor tends to reduce the distance over-target of inner London Health Districts but is not used by all the Thames Regions currently. The GLC justifies its case for taking social deprivation into account in RAWP, including a weighting for the social class composition and the proportion of one parent families, by reference to DOE'S analysis of the 1981 Census which shows that Inner London is one of the most deprived parts of England and Wales.

In the late 1970s, Forsyth and Varley (1981) carried out an analysis of the interaction of the Inner City Partnerships aimed at concentrating resources on specific parts of certain inner cities, with the policies being implemented by their corresponding NHS authorities, which were diverting resources elsewhere. Inner city health authorities were only able to fund developments in the priority services by schemes to reduce the number of acute beds, which in turn were dependent either on being able to make more intensive use of the remaining beds or to transfer a proportion of care into the community. However this process was seen to be inhibited by the inadequacy of local GP services, by poor housing conditions to discharge patients to and by opposition to closures and rationalisation, from consultants, trade unions and CHCs. Faced with these limitations on their room for manoeuvre, AHAs tended to try and use Inner City Partnership and Joint Funding as a development fund for the priority services at a time of restricted growth.

The basic problem in the implementation of RAWP and Partnership schemes stemmed from a conflict between the policies of DOE and DHSS at central government level. Health authority revenue allocations were to be reduced as the population migrated away from the inner cities, while Inner City Partnership arrangements had as one of their objectives to halt and reverse population decline in the same localities. Forsyth and Varley noted that the NHS planned according to OPCS population projections which assumed continued out-migration from the cities, despite the existence by then of Government policies to limit New Town growth and discontinue overspill developments (Forsyth and Varley, 1981, p.57).

At local level, AHAs with Partnerships found it 'virtually impossible to meet the Partnership requirement to redirect their expenditure towards the Partnership districts'. Other difficulties arose because of the different financial and administrative structure and organisation of health and local authorities. More fundamentally, the existence of Partnerships revealed conflicts in the local criteria for deciding priorities for funding. Partnership initiatives were intended to increase employment in the inner cities and reverse the pattern of selective out-migration. Health policies aimed at reducing the number of acute beds, had a contrary effect in that large city centre hospitals were a major source of employment for local people. However, Partnerships tended to concentrate on industrial and commercial employment development, largely ignoring the potential of the NHS. Another conflict of outlook identified by Forsyth and Varley was the unwillingness of Partnerships to accept for funding, schemes such as those in the NHS in which access was open to people from outside the Partnership area, thus failing to grasp the nature of cross-boundary flows in the NHS (Forsyth and Varley, 1981, pp.60-61).

RAWP's Treatment of Cross-Boundary Flows

RAWP recommended methods for RHAs which compensate for acute inpatient flows for revenue targets and ignore those in capital targets. No systematic attempt was made to distinguish between patient movements which were the result of convenience and those made from necessity. In deciding revenue targets RAWP made no reference to the possible usefulness of discriminating between flows which ought to continue because authority boundaries do not match the "natural" catchments of hospitals and those which ought to stop because they reflect a maldistribution of facilities (Bevan, 1982a, p.10). The system as it stands makes it difficult to decide which flows should be eliminated and over what timescale. RAWP considered that the need to discriminate between patient flows would be dealt with through the implementation of capital RAWP and the deployment of adequate capital resources in each locality to ensure equal access to hospitals by patients. When allocating capital to AHAs/Districts it was recognised that 'RHAs would need to take account of those cross-boundary patient flows which RHAs consider desirable' (DHSS, 1976c, p.70). At Regional level, RAWP's use of existing cross-boundary flows as a given in calculating revenue targets is of limited practical importance (except perhaps between the four Thames Regions) because the adjustments for flows is small compared with the remainder of the target derived from the residential population of a Region. However, sub-Regionally, particularly for inner city Districts, it is a critical matter since allowances for cross-boundary flows form a major element in District targets. The technical arguments about compensating for flows in targets are reviewed in Chapter Six. Here the literature on how flows are planned strategically and DHA responses to RHA reallocation policies is reviewed.

Planning Flows and District Self-Sufficiency

Butts reviewed the first round of Regional Strategic Plans in 1981 and highlighted patient flow calculations as 'crucial in determining the levels and siting of future services...' (Butts et al, 1981, p.95), yet each of the four Thames Regions was using a different method of calculation for RAWP purposes and for making assumptions about future flows for strategic planning. The London Health Planning Consortium made different assumptions again about patient flows. The Consortium assumed that the pattern of flows could not easily be changed but did not consider the implications for resource allocation policy of its analysis (LHPC, 1979 and 1980). It is apparent in a conurbation where there are no definite demographic boundaries, that a key strategic planning issue is to define and enumerate the population on behalf of which an administrative District is to plan and develop services in detail and to which a Region can allocate resources (Forsyth and Varley, 1981, p.54). This requires, however, that resource allocation and planning processes are integrated in recognition of their interrelationship, which is not easy to achieve within the current framework. It also requires an understanding and resolution of the difficulties which the notion of District "self-sufficiency" has created for planning health services in cities in relation to patient flows.

Preoccupations with self-sufficiency can be traced to three developments in the 1970s: firstly, the ambiguous statements in the 1974 reorganisation documents concerning the statutory responsibility of Area Health Authorities to ensure that their populations had access to a comprehensive range of health services (DHSS, 1972a); secondly, the way in which the broad objective and methods in the RAWP Report of equal opportunity of access to health care for people at equal risk were misinterpreted by managers (DHSS, 1976c, p.7, para. 1.3); thirdly, the emphasis since 1974 on "coterminosity" of Health Authorities with the relevant local authorities which often required the drawing of administrative boundaries with no real thought to the catchments of existing hospitals (Forsyth and Varley, 1981, p.54). Perrin et al (Royal Commission on the National Health Service, 1978a, p.29, para. B5.6) noted a tendency for both AHAs and Districts to favour self-sufficiency. Areas commonly mistook their statutory responsibility to plan a comprehensive health service for one of providing this service for the Area. The 1976 RAWP Report discouraged the notion:

'Total self-sufficiency in every AHA and District is not an immediate or necessarily even a longer-term aim.'
(DHSS, 1976c, p.43, para. 3.16)

Yet it would be unwise to assume that AHA officers read and digested even half the welter of information, advice and instructions which were sent to them in the relatively hectic period following the 1974 reorganisation! RAWP was often mistakenly assumed to have supported the notion of self-sufficiency. The DHSS tried subsequently on a number of occasions to discourage rigid notions of self-sufficiency. For example, DHSS Planning Guidelines for 1978-79 stated:

'...the objective of making local provision for comprehensive health care...does not necessarily imply that AHAs and Health Districts should aim at total self-sufficiency in the normal range of hospital specialities within their administrative boundaries, but rather at equality of opportunity of access to services...Planners must distinguish between cross-boundary flows of patients which are "natural" in a geographical sense and acceptable, and those which are distorted by present imbalances in the location of specialist services which their strategic planning must set out to correct.'
(quoted in Royal Commission on the National Health Service, 1978a, p.30, para. B5.8)

But such exhortation is unlikely to counteract the tendency it is intended to correct because of the difficulty of distinguishing between "natural" and other flows and the political pressures for District self-sufficiency. In the mid and late 1970s, Health Service planners were only slowly growing accustomed to rational, needs-based, notions of planning and to drawing up plans which were not predicated on assumptions of real growth in NHS resources at the rate which had prevailed in the late 1960s. The tendency remained to think incrementally about service developments and this contributed to the implicit objective of AHA/District self-sufficiency. In a period of ample growth in NHS funds this would have posed few problems, but when resources were sharply constrained it could have inefficient consequences. Perrin and colleagues noted the danger of over-provision and waste resulting from plans based on self-sufficiency, particularly in the Thames Regions (Royal Commission on the National Health Service, 1978a, p.30, para. B5.10). Forsyth and Varley noted similar pressures on the Regions covering the Manchester and Birmingham conurbations to plan on the basis of <u>predicted</u> population shifts and to build DGHs in the districts surrounding their city centres, even when there was easy access from the suburbs to existing hospitals (Forsyth and Varley, 1981, p.55).

Perhaps notions of "civic pride" and mistaken analogies with the role of local authorities vis-a-vis their residents also lie behind these pressures. Before the RAWP report was published, Buxton and Klein (1975) had queried the wisdom of health authorities modelled on local authorities when it came to sub-Regional resource allocation:

> 'Why have such an authority [Area Health Authority] if its boundaries do not make sense in terms of the distribution of health care resources but are the by-product...of local government reorganization whose logic (if any) is not necessarily the logic of health care provision?...While most local authorities are self-sufficient, whatever the level of the services they provide, the same is not true of many AHAs.'

Additionally, no doubt there is a stimulus to self-sufficiency from the fact that managers would prefer to have direct control over the services which are being provided for patients who are residents within their administrative boundaries rather than having to rely on other authorities for information on whether care was satisfactory or not. In turn, most health authority members tend to identify the interests of the authority with those of the local community.

However, there are incentives towards self-sufficiency within the actual methods of RAWP itself as they impinge on DHAs (Bevan, 1984). For Districts required to reduce expenditure to meet RAWP targets there is a short-term incentive to refuse referrals of residents from other Districts. This is only an expedient since such action will in turn result in deductions from the District's target and eventually a reduction in the District's budget. Fox (1978, pp.45-7) noted that the assumption in RAWP that transfer prices should not be adjusted for case complexity but should be at the average cost per specialty, introduced incentives particularly for teaching districts with large cross-boundary flows, which could distort decisions on who to treat and which health service to consider a high priority. He perceptively detected emerging trends at an early stage:

> '...some districts, faced with limited resources, have already started to favour their own residents, often by keeping non-residents on the waiting-list longer. This practice may not be public knowledge, or even explicit policy. Rather, the hospital doctor is made to understand that he has a moral obligation to serve district residents first.'
> (Fox, 1978, p.46)

In 1985 Camberwell Health Authority banned patients who live outside the District from receiving routine treatment at its hospitals in a misguided effort to improve its position relative to its target (Feinmann, 1985). An official of the Authority was quoted as commenting on the decision as follows:

'"But quite frankly, I don't see why we should treat bunions for the fat cats in Hastings and Bexhill-on-Sea"'.

Similar policies have been discussed in a number of other inner London Districts such as Bloomsbury and West Lambeth.

Bevan (1984) points to a second incentive to eliminate cross-boundary flows experienced by Districts wishing to have control over their long-term RAWP position. Authorities cannot prevent referrals of their residents for treatment in other Districts, yet this results in them having a lower RAWP target and a lower budget. This creates pressure to improve their target position by trying to limit the scale of referrals outside the District, either by attempting directly to influence the choices of GPs and patients about hospitals, or by attempting to invest in facilities which will attract residents. This latter approach to self-sufficiency through supplying further beds, can lead to practical problems. Since supply fuels demand, an increase in District bed numbers to prevent outflows of residents may fail to stem the outflows but may attract more patients from outside the District.

Greenshields (1984, p.1394), then a Regional Treasurer, put the self-sufficient preoccupations of some urban Districts into perspective:

'In the present financial climate we must be sure that all resources are being used to achieve the greatest value for money. Part of that exercise must be to maximise the return from present investment in building stock, a policy that may lead to some district services being provided on behalf of other districts in many instances. This may be unfortunate but it is a short to medium term necessity. When present capital stock requires replacing, however, it is imperative to replace it in the appropriate location for the population to be served.'

Greenshields is implicitly advocating a close tie between planning and resource allocation. Where he talks of the greatest 'value for money' in the current jargon, others might prefer "efficiency", since blocking admissions from outside administrative boundaries of Districts may well lead to an inefficient use of NHS resources. It is also inequitable, since patients who faced long waiting times in their District of residence, which may well be the result of historically low levels of provision, would be prevented from going to other Districts with shorter waiting times. Given the huge variations in waiting times around the country (Anonymous, 1985) there would seem to be a need to facilitate a flexible pattern of referrals and to view the NHS as an integrated, national system rather than to erect barriers. The College of Health has been trying to do this through its Guide to Hospital Waiting Lists (College of Health, 1985).

It would appear from Camberwell's example, that a potentially important policy decision about the balance between equity and efficiency goals in the NHS was taken unplanned by one District as a short-run response to the perceived demands of the RAWP process to reduce expenditure. In addition, it is probable that the District was concerned about the cost of its inflows and whether or not these were adequately compensated for in the RAWP target calculation (see Chapter Six for a discussion of this issue). Thus in a direct way, the technicalities of RAWP can be seen shaping policies over which patient flows should remain and which should be terminated, with no reference to the overall Regional situation. Similar, discriminatory policies against "out-of-District" patients are emerging in a number of other RAWP-losing Districts with potentially serious consequences in terms of equity and the notion of a National Health Service.

On a more general level, a mechanical formula through which a District's projected allocations depend on the build-up of the components of its target, including its catchment population, rather than approval of its plans or past performance in matching plans to actual expenditure, provides no financial incentive for local managers to implement DHSS priorities (Varley, 1982). There is, on the contrary, a danger that planning decisions will be taken on the basis of their impact on RAWP targets and subsequent allocations. In inner-cities, cross-boundary flows are very significant and boundaries are meaningless for acute services. Thus a method which starts from the residential population and then tries to adjust for cross-boundary flows would seem inappropriate. In such situations, reductions in expenditure may also reduce the RAWP target, thus the District has an incentive to work out in detail the components of its target and to model what effect different patterns of reduction in expenditure will have on the target. Although this may be a rational exercise for the District, it violates a basic RAWP principle that the target should never become the basis for policy, since it is generated from past patterns of expenditure.

INTEGRATION OF PLANNING AND RESOURCE ALLOCATION SUB-REGIONALLY

In response to the difficulties of using RAWP sub-Regionally and of reconciling its demands with the needs of the planning process, RHAs have exploited their relative autonomy in resource allocation to make a variety of modifications to the formulation of RAWP targets and the process for allocating resources. Some of this work is contained in unpublished documents produced for internal Regional consumption - some in Strategic Plans and other public documents; but little or none of it has entered the published literature. In certain Regions, even senior District Managers are not privy to the intricacies of the methods of sub-Regional allocation. Thus the description which follows is inevitably incomplete. A detailed, up-to-date review of Regional activities in this field is not available, but would be a useful aide-memoire for policy-makers now that RAWP has been in existence for a decade. In addition a number of commentators have identified possible alternative models for use in resource allocation by RHAs and have recommended formal changes to RAWP. These are described below.

Modifications by Regions to the Method of Calculating Targets

There are opportunities to modify the mechanics of the RAWP formula itself to relate it more closely to Regional planning priorities without going as far as the full integration of resource allocation and planning. A survey of all RHAs in 1982 carried out by the National Association of Health Authorities (NAHA) concluded that every Region had found it necessary to modify the RAWP methodology, but only one Region claimed to be using an entirely different methodology (National Association of Health Authorities, 1983, para.4). The majority admitted to no formal mechanism for reconciling resource allocation with planning (NAHA, 1983 para. 18) despite the fact that various methods had been discussed in certain RHAs for some time (e.g. Morris, 1979).
The main formula modifications with planning implications which have taken place in some Regions are:

1. use of relative expenditure proportions in the service categories of the revenue formula which reflect planning guidelines or the content of RHA and DHA plans rather than historical expenditure proportions (Butts et al, 1981, pp. 171-172);

2. use of current population estimates or even population projections rather than past data (Abel-Smith, 1981, p.58);

3. recasting of mental illness and mental handicap elements in the formula (all RHAs) (e.g. by basing components on a weighted catchment population) including removing these services from RAWP altogether (National Association of Health Authorities, 1983, para. 11);

4. funding Regional specialties by "top-slicing" or on the basis of the demands made on such services by each District (Bevan and Spencer, 1984, p.106);

5. use of catchment populations rather than resident populations with a separate cross-boundary flow adjustment, as a base for the non-psychiatric inpatient services target; or targets based on projected patient flows expected to result from planning changes (e.g. closures); or use of catchment populations based on geographical access measured by travelling time (Butts et al, 1981, p.169);

6. inclusion of allowances for outpatient and daypatient cross-boundary flows;

7. compensating certain cross-boundary flows at an estimate of actual cost rather than national average specialty costs.

Approaches to Resource Allocation Sub-Regionally

The RAWP Report recommended that the pace of movement towards revenue targets at AHA and District level should be determined not by rigid 'floors' and 'ceilings', but flexibly, by discussion between the tiers of management with due regard to local factors and planning considerations such as the need to develop priority services, decisions on patterns of care and consequent patient flows and decisions on "centres of excellence" (DHSS, 1976c, p.44, para. 3.16). Had these recommendations been developed subsequently by DHSS in the form of guidance to Regions, it is possible that a far more integrated approach to resource allocation and planning could have been instituted sub-Regionally. However, from the analysis of planning and resource allocation since 1976 in this Chapter, it would seem that RHAs tended to adopt a fairly rigid, target-led approach to financial allocations based on variants of the RAWP formula, particularly in the early days after 1976/77. Since then, Regions have developed a variety of approaches to setting goals of equity sub-Regionally. Bevan and Spencer (1984) identified four models of Regional resource policy current in the early 1980s along a continuum from considerable local autonomy to strong Regional direction:

1. Devolved financial - the approach of national RAWP in which targets for capital and revenue and the pace of movement to targets are decided separately by independent formulae.

2. Revenue-led - revenue allocations are mainly decided on the principle of reducing the variation around revenue targets. Thus revenue dominates resource policy.

3. Capital-led - capital allocations are mainly decided on the principle of reducing the variation around capital targets. The region funds the RCCS (Revenue Consequences of Capital Schemes). Thus, the funding of RCCS is the main influence on revenue allocations to Districts.

4. Planning-based - decisions to build new hospitals and other facilities are taken on the basis of a review of services carried out as part of the planning process rather than through comparison with capital targets. This review enables a schedule of Districts' priorities to be drawn up and capital is allocated to fund the schedule. The Region funds the RCCS which

is the main influence on revenue allocations of Districts. Thus, planning
is the motor of changes in resource policy.
(Bevan and Spencer, 1984, p.109)

Bevan and Spencer argue that devolved target-based methods (1.-3. above) have a
number of common weaknesses, notably, the fact that in critical locations (e.g.
inner city teaching Districts) the reliability of targets as a basis for policy
is in doubt (because of statistical adjustments) and that since the method of
calculating targets is not derived from a coherent set of strategic objectives
it cannot provide a sound basis for major resource shifts. Yet, the majority of
Regions' efforts have gone towards responding to demands from Districts for
refinements of various detailed aspects of their Regional RAWP formulae, rather
than the more difficult task of integrating RAWP with the planning system.

However, since the late 1970s a few Regions have discussed, piloted and some
have partially implemented, resource allocation methods which attempt to
integrate resource allocation and planning sub-Regionally. Whitt reports that
in 1978, Oxford RHA was actively considering using its strategic plan as an
alternative basis for revenue funding and that West Midlands RHA piloted an
'Integrated Planning and Resource Allocation System' in 1980-81, in which a
proportion of Regional revenue was to be allocated by RAWP and the remainder in
response to Area plans (Butts et al, 1981, p.178 and Morris, 1979).   However,
West Midlands RHA had still not implemented a fully integrated system by the
time of the NAHA survey in 1982. Capital allocations were determined in
accordance with the priorities in the strategic plan, but RAWP revenue targets
were not reconciled with service planning and there was no retrospective
comparison between target and actual expenditure for particular services (NAHA,
1983).   Indeed, by the time of the NAHA survey, despite considerable discussion
of methods (e.g. Morris, 1979) only Wessex and Yorkshire RHAs were explicitly
claiming to have evolved an integrated approach to planning and resource
allocation. The Wessex methodology for revenue was the only one at that time to
be portrayed by its authors as marking a complete departure from a RAWP-type
approach. The target was replaced by a 'Revenue Goal' for each District and
care group, based on planned standards of provision which established the notion
of "like resources for like populations".   The object was to achieve revenue
equity within 15 years by attaining the 'Revenue Goal'. Movement towards equity
was determined by an annual distribution related to each District's distance
from its 'Revenue Goal'. Implicit in the approach was the reconciliation of
resource allocation and service planning. However, the method of calculating
the 'Revenue Goal' was not reported in the NAHA Survey (NAHA, 1983, paras. 4-5).
Although the detailed methodology has not been made available even to Districts
within Wessex, it is possible to infer the outline from planning documents. The
revenue goal is calculated on the basis of norms of provision ('Service
Standards') (e.g. numbers of acute beds per 1,000 population) which generate
the need for levels of direct care and support staff derived from staffing norms
('Manpower Standards') (e.g. numbers of whole-time equivalents per bed).   The
number of staff required to maintain the level of provision indicated by the
norms, is then converted into financial terms and this is the 'revenue goal'
(Wessex RHA, 1984).

The methodology for capital involved a similar process based on establishing
normative 'goals' for each District and care group and establishing an
'Investment Framework' designed to equalise the relative position over time.

Since the NAHA survey (1982) it would seem that a number of Regions are now
developing revenue allocation approaches based on funding agreed District plans
rather than using a RAWP-type approach, although it is not possible to obtain a
detailed account of exactly how each of these procedures operates (Greenshields,
1984, p. 1394). For example, North Western RHA has developed a service-based
approach to resource allocation within a care group framework in which 'service

targets' influence but do not determine allocations, and growth monies coming to the Region through national RAWP are distributed to Districts via a bidding process according to national priorities. South West and North West Thames RHAs have both recently decided to depart from formal use of a sub-Regional formula. From the financial year 1985/86 the allocation of resources to Districts will be determined by the Regional Strategic Plan, although the Plans themselves have been influenced by RAWP-type methods (GLC Health Panel, 1984, p.15). However, there is no published summary of the current situation sub-Regionally.

A number of writers have concluded that sub-Regionally, the planning system is a more suitable basis for allocating resources than even the most sophisticated top-down formula, particularly for hospital services (Mullen, 1978, p. 25; Butts and Ashford, 1977). Greenshields argues from his experience in North Western RHA that:

> 'putting agreed health care aims first and the fair allocation of the available funds to support them as a follow on....seems to be the correct sequence. This approach also provides a fairer basis for distribution of resources by allowing for the levels of health care to be provided and the levels of efficiency to be achieved by districts in that provision.' (Greenshields, 1984, p.1394)

It may be objected that the planning-based model looks similar to the pre-1974, if not pre-1971, model of resource allocation with the risk that equitable solutions will be prejudiced by competition from attractive and powerfully-supported schemes favouring the "haves" rather than the "have nots". Since there are no published accounts of the effects on equity of a planning-based model in practice, it is impossible to say. However, where the planning-based approach differs from the pre-1974 model is in the important fact that capital and in turn revenue developments are supposedly drawn from a system of service planning which did not exist previously (Bevan and Spencer, 1984, p.110). In addition, in a period of very limited or nil growth in NHS resources, a planning-based approach recommends itself, since it requires explicit choices to be made about where, how and with what priority, resources should be committed to different parts of the health system.

Suggested Models of Integrating Planning and Resource Allocation

The literature on RAWP sadly contains virtually nothing which describes RHAs' attempts to integrate planning and resouce allocation. This is a most significant omission as RHAs are developing fast in this direction with no outside comment on their approaches or ability easily to compare RHA practice. In this section there is no alternative but to rely on what is largely speculation about what might be done.

The first model was proposed by Butts and Ashford (1977) who aimed to provide a practical, planning-based alternative to RAWP for acute hospital services. The authors describe in some detail a hospital planning methodology which enables need for services to be estimated and translated into requirements for hospital beds and other resources at District level. They then describe how a RHA may best fulfil its prime function of controlling resource distribution between AHAs and Districts by harmonising the 'planning scenarios' for each District (e.g. by ensuring that resource usage rates are equalised over a defined period) and funding these scenarios accordingly. The allocation of capital and revenue is viewed as an integral part of such systematic planning. Current and planned future resource requirements are converted into financial resources for each District and by specialty for in-patients and out-patients, using a statistical technique to derive average Regional Specialty costs based on the linkage of SH3 returns to standard Hospital Cost Returns. This process yields current and future notional revenue estimates for each District which can then be expressed as percentages of the Region's total allocation to allow the actual subdivision of the Region's allocation. Advantages of this method are held to be that:

1. It is superior to the normative approach.

2. Planned <u>local</u> utilization rates are used implicitly in preference to national rates to reflect local needs.

3. Resource calculations are based on routine Regional data and link coherently with planning assumptions.

4. Allocations would not give extra money to specialties costing more than the Regional average (i.e. an incentive to seek out inefficiencies).

5. The method is not incremental and represents an escape from "last year's budget plus x per cent".

The process described by Butts and Ashford (1977) presumes a critical role for Regional Health Authorities in ensuring, through discussion and negotiation, that the assumptions and 'planning scenarios' adopted by different localities in the Region are mutually consistent. The Regions also have an important role in providing analyses of the extensive routine SH3 and HAA data required for the planning and resource allocation process. Butts and Ashford justified making no special allowances for above-average costs in particular specialties on the basis that investigations had failed to account for the observed cost variations between Districts and that each District or AHA would have a range of hospitals and specialties between the extremes of high and low unit costs. This approach appears simplistic in the light of subsequent debates about the reasons for the justification of the differential costs of hospitals with different case-mixes and the recent use of Diagnosis Related Groups as a basis for costing case-mix (Bevan, 1982b; Maxwell, 1984; Culyer, Wiseman, Drummond and West, 1978; Dredge, 1984; Jenkins and Coles, 1984).

Morris (1979) proposed a straightforward approach to reconciling planning priorities and spatial inequality. In his proposed approach, an AHA's Operational Plan would contain five-year capital, revenue and manpower projections which would become its resource allocation submission in year 1 and its capital bid for future years. Authorities would also obtain a development addition (or deduction) made up of two parts: a guaranteed basic sum depending on distance from RAWP target and a supplementary addition according to an AHA's progress towards achieving agreed planning priorities. The same procedure would apply to capital and revenue allocations. Apart from basic allocations, the remainder of an AHA's allocation would be dependent upon compatibility with agreed planning priorities. Conformity with priorities would be monitored by the RHA by reference to changes in client group expenditure and manpower patterns. If an AHA did not, over a period, devote resources to the objectives to which they had originally been assigned, the RHA would make an appropriate deduction in the AHA's future allocation. Morris (1979) perceived the system to have a number of advantages:

1. A positive relationship between planning and resource allocation was built into the system which provides incentives for authorities to produce thorough, realistic plans in line with priorities.

2. The move towards spatial equity should become less mechanistic.

3. Capital and revenue allocations would be seen to be interrelated.

4. Regional specialties would be treated no differently from other service developments.

5. A framework for subsequent monitoring would be provided.

Possible problems were seen to be:

1. The planning system was insufficiently developed to bear the burden of resource allocation.

2. Techniques were not yet available to calculate the cost of planning intentions in sufficient detail.

3. The system would alter the relationship between RHAs and AHAs/Districts.

4. It would be difficult to penalise an authority for not following agreed priorities by reducing its subsequent allocations.

A problem which Morris did not discuss is the possibility with such a planning-based system that the desired budget for a Region (based on 'target' District service levels, at, say, DHSS specialty costs) would exceed its actual allocation!

In a recent text-book on National Health Service finance, Jones and Prowle (1984, pp. 34-37, 46-48, 100-104) provide perhaps the most extended discussion of resource allocation methods. They outline three alternatives to RAWP: capital-led revenue allocations; revenue allocations derived from annual programmes (plans); and DRG costing. In relation to planning, they describe a theoretical system for resource allocation to both RHAs and DHAs using the NHS planning system which is similar to the methods used by the Department of The Environment for resource allocation with reference to local authority transport and housing programmes. They observe that capital and revenue allocation is a powerful planning and priority implementation tool not currently used to the full in the NHS, because of a prior commitment both to geographical equity through RAWP and a devolved structure which allows the periphery considerable autonomy in the use of resources. For revenue allocations to DHAs by Regions, Jones and Prowle envisage a process in which resources would be distributed in the form of development additions as long as DHA strategic plans and annual programmes have been judged to be in conformity with national policies and priorities. Resources would not necessarily be earmarked, nor would the amount of the development addition necessarily be derived from the additional cost of the particular proposal it related to, but the allocation would be built up from approved plans. It would be a recognition that the projects proposed had the general support of the Secretary of State. (However, there seems no reason with increasingly sophisticated budgeting and costing methods, why development additions should not derive directly from particular proposals.) For capital, they envisage a similar system for large schemes, with a block grant for smaller schemes (perhaps on a RAWP basis) and a monitoring system to check that allocations have been used for their proper purpose.

However, Jones and Prowle appear to reject such a planning-based approach for use by DHSS for allocations to Regions on the grounds that in their view it fails a test of their three principles of resource allocation - equity, objectivity and simplicity. (It is not clear how these three principles were chosen ahead of possible alternatives.) They feel that such a method may work for allocations by Regions to DHAs; although they seem pessimistic about the prospects for limiting opportunism and wheeling and dealing. This may be partly because they do not consider the likely changes in RHA-DHA relations and patterns of Regional influence which would be required if a planning-based approach were to be implemented. At the same time, they overestimate the "objectivity" of RAWP in terms of its ability to stand outside the political arena of the NHS. They presume that the current RAWP process is immune from political influence and that the rules of the game are clearly and publicly defined, making covert political bargaining impossible. Part of the problem in their analysis may be due to a failure to distinguish clearly enough between the procedure for formulating RAWP targets and the process of making actual allocations: the former may be regarded as insulated to an extent, from political pressures, whereas the latter is much less so.

Jones and Prowle propose a system of District programme budgeting which provides the means both of planning and monitoring the attainment of objectives and priorities. Theoretically, this should increase the likelihood of plans being implemented (Mooney, 1984; Mooney, Russell and Weir, 1980, pp.63-75). The principal advantages of the system are:

1. It would combine resource allocation with planning and enable DHSS and Regions to consider both geographical equity and care group priorities in deciding allocations.

2. Planning would become more effective because it would become the means to attract resources and this would be an incentive to improve the quality of planning.

Jones and Prowle claim that such a system imposes a number of healthy requirements on the NHS which are not met by current arrangements:

1. It would require a considerable development in financial information systems so that a detailed revenue programme showing how monies are and will be spent by care group can be drawn up.

2. Authorities would have to change from functional to care group accounting.

3. Authorities would have to submit spending programmes within resource assumptions; thus, the secretary of State would have to express a firm view on future growth in NHS resources.

4. Controls and monitoring devices would need to be devised to ensure that money was spent on schemes put forward in plans and financial programmes.

Jones and Prowle note the possible disadvantages of the system:

1. Such a procedure could be susceptible to political influence and this could result in a reinforcement of the current skewed distribution of health resources.

2. If the sum available for development additions were less than anticipated, RHAs, would have to rank DHA proposals in priority order and allocate resources in sequence, but this process too could be susceptible to political influence by DHAs.

3. The system would tend to ignore geographical inequalities in favour of client group inequalities (it is not clear why Jones and Prowle exclude the possibility that considerations of geographical equity cannot be built into the planning process and why client group priorities should always take precedence in this process).

4. An objective comparison between RHAs and DHAs may not be possible because authorities may use different data bases and have different definitions of need.

5. The process would make resource allocation much more complicated.

Further discussion of some of the points raised by Jones and Prowle is given in the concluding chapter of this review.

While Jones and Prowle broadly prefer the RAWP approach at national level they discuss alternatives to RAWP other than use of the planning system, particularly for use in determining allocations to DHAs. They also consider possible combinations of methods, since at present not all funds are "RAWPed" and District allocations commonly include the Service Increment for Teaching (SIFT), allowances for Regional specialties, other earmarked sums and Joint Finance. For allocating revenue they consider an old and a new method: capital-led resource allocation (i.e. funding the Revenue Consequences of Capital Schemes); and the use of Diagnosis Related Groups. They conclude that capital-led resource allocation is inadequate on its own since it only forms part of a comprehensive system for allocating resources, but that this weakness can be overcome by using it as a component in the planning-led methodology. Since Jones and Prowle's is a recent text (1984) they are able to sketch the possible uses of the American-originated concept of Diagnosis Related Groups (DRGs) for resource allocation. (Fetter, Shin, Freeman, Averill and Thompson, 1980; May, 1982). Since DRGs provide a way of classifying hospital patients into clusters broadly homogeneous in terms of resource use, the simplest way to use them for funding hospitals, according to Jones and Prowle, would be to multiply the planned number of patients in each DRG by the budgeted cost per patient for each DRG. The authors suggest a range of major obstacles to the use of DRGs for determining allocations from Regions to Districts in the NHS. Aside from technical problems of data, the DRG method has two main drawbacks as a method of integrating planning and resource allocation: firstly, DRGs apply only to hospital inpatient services; and secondly, they represent essentially a "bottom-up", demand-led approach, ignoring the fact that DHAs are cash-limited and that rationing theoretically takes place around national priorities based on need. With DRGs in the USA, resources are presumed to be made available on the basis of the number of patients requiring treatment. The use of DRGs in this fashion, to determine even a proportion of resources allocated in the NHS could endanger the development of the adequately funded community care and priority services by reinforcing the status quo in favour of acute services. On the other hand, there would appear to be no reason why the acute caseload of a District or hospital could not be agreed in advance, within certain limits through a planned approach and funded accordingly using DRGs. This would make it possible to work within a cash limit. However, the conclusion of Jones and Prowle (1984) and others who have looked at the potential application of DRGs in the British context is that although DRGs may have considerable merit for planning and as performance indicators, the circumstances of the NHS are not favourable to their use for resource allocation (Beech, Bevan and Brazier, 1985).

On the capital side, Jones and Prowle (1984) are clear that allocations to major schemes should be determined through the planning system rather than through any formula-based approach. For minor capital allocations (however defined), they note the variety of procedures in use by Regions but do not express any preferences except to say that RAWP-type population methods are inappropriate for capital (something RHAs appreciated as soon as RAWP was introduced) and that attention should be given to the, as yet untried, 'bidding approach' described as an option in the 1976 RAWP Report (DHSS, 1976c, pp.133-4, paras. E1-E5).

Unlike most other writers in this field, Jones and Prowle suggest permutations of the main four approaches (RAWP-type, capital-led, planning-led and DRG costing) for use by RHAs which would reduce some of the problems of political influence and 'subjectivity' which they perceive in the planning-based approach.

An example would be for a Region to "top-slice" funds earmarked to the priority care groups and distribute these monies in pursuance of DHA annual programmes, with the remainder of the Region's funds allocated by RAWP principles. Any development addition coming to the Region could be used partly to finance RCCS, with the remainder to be allocated by RAWP principles. In some ways, this is comparable to current practice in a number of Regions. However, they conclude by rescuing the planning-led approach:

'Our assessment is that revenue allocations based on annual programmes will probably be the most appropriate method in most regions. It would fit all the criteria above [viz. 1. sensitive to regional circumstances, 2. Based on a generally acceptable measurement of need, 3. explicit, 4. comprehensive] and in particular because it would be based on regionally provided information, it would be particularly sensitive to the DHAs' requirements... Furthermore it would substantially overcome the criticism...about the lack of reconciliation between planning and resource allocation.'
(Jones and Prowle, 1984, p.105)

Bevan and Spencer (1984) have also considered new ways of formulating resource policies, specifically for acute hospital services, since they consider that RAWP crucially fails to offer a strategic basis for resource allocation and a coordinated way of making changes at District level. Their most important criticism is that sub-Regional RAWP fails to relate decisions about resources to the planned need for services. As a means of enabling those responsible better to understand the links between decisions on financial allocations, plans and services, for the acute sector, they describe in outline a tentative approach still under development, based on the catchment populations of individual acute specialties. The method essentially provides a way of assessing the extent of relative overprovision and resource deprivation in acute hospital resources between Districts, based on workload. It suggests possible alternative dispositions of services to remedy imbalances (using a gravity model of flows to hospitals) and expresses the likely costs and benefits of options for changing the location of beds and related services. The method would assess under-provision or over-provision by applying the Regional average rate of hospitalisation by age and sex for each specialty to the population of each District. This would give a case-load norm which could be compared to the actual number of residents treated whether in the District or elsewhere. The extent of the difference would provide an indicator of over-provision or under-provision which could be adjusted to reflect available evidence of differences in morbidity.

A second, similar method of hospital resource allocation is discussed in more recent work by the same author (Bevan, 1984). The method is again based on using relative hospitalisation rates (ie. cases treated) as indicators of "need" for, or under-provision of, services. In essence the approach would relate funding of hospitals to financial targets based on cases treated, determined by GP referrals rather than a weighted residential population as in RAWP. In order not to perpetuate inequalities in provision between Districts, incentives to promote more equal access would be built into the system by taking account of whether cases came from Districts with ralatively high or low hospitalisation rates. Cases from Districts with high hospitalisation rates would contribute less to a hospital's target than cases from so-called "deprived" Districts thus providing incentives for over-provided Districts to treat patients from under-provided Districts. Workload targets could be set for hospitals and Districts as part of strategic planning exercises to make the distribution of capital and revenue more equal.

An obvious problem with the first method as described (Bevan and Spencer, 1984) is its reliance on the assumption that specialties contain a similar case-mix in different Districts. However, the development of DRGs for use in Britain may well provide an improved description of case-mix for this purpose. This method would continue to allocate resources for community-based services using a RAWP-type population-based approach. The second method (Bevan, 1984) also requires a more detailed classification of case-mix than the conventional specialties will allow and DRGs could be used in this case. It also requires a more accurate method than is currently available for costing cross-boundary flow cases.

CONCLUSIONS

This chapter has drawn attention to the problems which the lack of integration of planning and resource allocation in the NHS has posed for the implementation sub-Regionally of policies designed to remedy care group and geographical deficiencies in health services. The majority of those who recognised this problem explicitly have chosen to abandon the RAWP formula in favour of some method of basing equitable resource allocation around a strategic analysis of how services should develop and be deployed. The extent of variation in resources sub-Regionally is such that even when in the 1990s Regions are on or near their RAWP targets, the need to redistribute resources within RHAs and between DHAs in neighbouring RHAs will remain.

In practice, of course, an unintended link has been forged between RAWP and planning because of the necessity to make trade-offs between geographical equity and care group priorities in a period of very restricted growth in resources. Hence, the pace of movement towards RAWP targets has been affected by other planning priorities especially in sub-Regional RAWP. Bosanquet (1980) in his review of the Labour Government's record in health policy, 1974-79, comments that by 1979 it was apparent that the metropolitan RHAs were applying redistribution extremely slowly because of political resistance and the perceived need to build up priority services in inner London. In recognition of this, for example, in 1979/80, London Regions were granted an extra 1% revenue growth (at the expense of slowing down the movement to RAWP target of the under-target Regions) to speed up the redistribution to the non-metropolitan parts of the four Thames Regions. At the same time, extra funds outside the RAWP process were also allocated by DHSS to some inner London Districts to improve their community health services in recognition of problems of social deprivation and poor GP services attested to in the Acheson Report (London Health Planning Consortium,1981).

It is precisely at District level in the inner cities, especially in London and the other conurbations, where there is a need for a consistent approach to resource allocation between adjacent Regions and Districts, because of the extent of cross-boundary flows. This chapter has shown in various ways that sub-Regional RAWP targets fail to provide good and reliable indicators in these circumstances of where money should be removed from certain Districts in order to finance services in less well-provided Regions and Districts. Historically this is because in the mid-1970s, when the RAWP methodology was conceived, inequality in the availability of health service resources between Regions was the main focus of concern. As a result, most of the thinking went into providing a method for financial allocations to Regions and at this level, RAWP appears to work reasonably successfully because of the relative homogeneity of populations.

The concept of redistribution and of equalising access geographically within the NHS is in danger of being discredited by the perversities of sub-Regional RAWP, particularly in those Districts in London which represent the "bank" for redistribution to the rest of the country and whose seemingly parochial concerns are of national significance. Stark inequalities in resource availability and resource consumption remain (DHSS, 1985a and 1986b) and will need to be addressed as long as the National Health Service's fundamental objectives remain in place. Thus, other means will have to be found to promote equity and to give Districts objectives which they can reasonably hope to attain. A number of Regions are beginning to appreciate these points and are developing ways of deriving DHA allocations from a Regional strategy, thus integrating resource allocation with planning. In this way, strategies have to be costed and realistic. The potential advantage of finance following from a process of Regional strategic management (apart from circumventing idiosyncracies of sub-Regional RAWP targets) is that since strategic plans are negotiated and agreed between tiers and since loser-Districts will be able to see exactly where resources are going and for what purpose, there will be more chance of generating the necessary commitment to redistribution and closures. A number of Regions are experimenting in this way, but it is difficult to obtain a coherent picture of the methods being used nor of their effects. There is a need therefore, to review Regional innovation in strategic management of financial allocations and service planning.

One logical way to apportion responsibilities in this context would be for the Region to be ultimately responsible (and accountable to DHSS) for the equitable distribution of services through a process of strategic management and for the Districts to be responsible for providing good quality services efficiently (Bevan and Brazier 1985b). District management would thus not be put in the difficult position of having to persuade Authority members to take the initiative themselves to cut acute services in an attempt to move towards (an often unattainable!) RAWP target.

In direct response to the difficulties encountered in implementing sub-Regional RAWP, North West Thames RHA has recently adopted a method of resource allocation based on Regional strategic management of change. Although only at an early stage, the approach may be indicative of one possible way forward. In developing a strategy for acute services the approach has been to examine how money could be made available for redistribution by rationalising the acute sector and what effect consequent changes in the number and distribution of hospital beds would have on equitable access to services across the Region (North West Thames RHA, 1984a). In this way it is hoped that closure decisions will reflect a strategic assessment of their impact primarily on equitable access (rather than Districts' solo attempts to meet their RAWP targets), but also taking into account factors such as clinical requirements of medical students and the quality of capital stock, which may be in conflict with equity. Under sub-Regional RAWP, Districts are given the problem of resolving these conflicts when they are not in a position to do so.

When a strategy has been hammered out for the phased redistribution of hospital acute services, DHA budgets will then derive from the strategy. In any given year, each District will have an expected number of beds and medical students, etc. Services will be funded on the basis of the expected caseload to be treated in each District given these numbers and assuming efficient use of beds. Allocations would be reduced or increased in a step-wise fashion to reflect the changes in provision indicated in the strategy (e.g. as wards or hospitals are opened and closed), rather than as often happens in sub-Regional RAWP, reduced or increased by a percentage rate each year, which may or may not accurately match changing provision requirements. A fuller discussion of the strategic management approach is contained in the concluding chapter.

It seems likely that explicit integration of resource allocation and planning processes would also entail major changes in relationships between tiers in the Health Service and would therefore have political costs. If it <u>were</u> to be attempted, one significant implication would be an enhanced role for RHAs as the tier of management in the NHS capable of reconciling the planning intentions of inter-related Districts and allocating resources accordingly. This would take as its starting point the existing role of Regions in strategic planning. Such a development would sit uneasily with the insistence in Patients First on 'the minimum of interference' from above in the affairs of Districts (DHSS, 1979, p.2) and run against the tone of the most recent priorities document, Care in Action (DHSS, 1981) which appears to envisage planning as dialogue, '...a continuing conversation between centre and periphery - as distinct from planning as command' (Klein, 1981, p.1090). It would imply an attempt to overcome some of the de facto decentralisation and local autonomy of the NHS which is based in the power of service providers, particularly the medical profession, to resist change. Several studies of local decision-making have suggested that centrally defined objectives frequently have limited impact at the periphery (Haywood and Alaszewski, 1980; Hunter, 1980; Ham, 1981). It would also reopen the long-running controversy within the NHS as to the appropriate balance between central direction and local responsiveness. It would probably be resisted by District management as a recipe for top-down bureaucracy and inflexibility, stifling local innovation and imagination and depriving local managers of the freedom to manage effectively in response to local wishes and circumstances.

However, seen from the point of view of attaining NHS objectives, the development of the Regional tier of the NHS appears to offer a valuable opportunity for:

1. District aspirations to be negotiated and reconciled with national policies and overall Regional considerations;

2. District plans to be approved and funded progressively within resource constraints;

3. a process of accountability review to be linked directly to resource allocation to assess whether or not policies are being implemented; and

4. future allocations to be contingent, at least in part, on attaining objectives in order to restrain the momentum of existing commitments.

The Royal Commission on the NHS recognised the potentially important strategic role of Regions and went as far as to recommend that RHAs should be directly accountable to Parliament for health service delivery (Royal Commission on the National Health Service, 1979, p.307, paras. 19.33 and 19.34). This was rejected politically, on the grounds that the incoming Conservative Government was at that time committed to strengthening clinical autonomy and devolving responsibility to the level at which services were actually delivered and constitutionally, on the grounds that since the NHS was centrally funded by the annual supply vote in Parliament, accountability could only be vested in the Secretary of State. However, the Royal Commission's recommendation found influential support more recently. The Griffiths Inquiry into NHS management identified the need to strengthen the role of Regions, particularly in planning, resource allocation and accountability review (DHSS, 1983, p.16, para.13).

Although the Government's emphasis since 1979 in policy documents concerning the structure of the NHS hierarchy, has been towards increasing District, unit and ultimately professional autonomy as much as possible; since 1981-82, concern to improve management and accountability in the Service has led to the development of a range of new tools for monitoring and performance review such as Performance Indicators and Regional Reviews. These tools would be of considerable value in developing an integrated system of planning and resource allocation steered from Regional level. It has been claimed that such systems need not necessarily consist of higher tiers imposing their will on a resistant periphery. Gray and Hunter (1983, pp.432-3) argue for the feasibility of a synthesis of "top-down" and "bottom-up" approaches to policy formulation, planning, resource allocation and implementation, requiring negotiation and information exchange between RHAs, DHAs and professionals, so that broad, often nebulous national statements of policy can be brought to the level of detail which makes sense at District and service delivery levels. However, they argue that the centre must be prepared to underpin such a process by defining what constitutes policy failure and what sanctions it is prepared to permit Regions to use if they are dissatisfied with what has happened in a District. They also make the important point that if change is genuinely to take place, the political and intellectual commitment to assessing plans and eventual resource deployment in relation to priorities must be sustained over a concerted period of time, since change in any one year will of necessity be marginal.

For the sort of system hinted at by Gray and Hunter to work more by negotiation than imposition, agreement has to be possible between Regions and Districts over objectives. In the main, conflict between Regions and Districts in the Health Service is fought out in terms of the means rather than the ends of policy, focusing on such matters as the pace of change and whether a particular policy has been adequately recognised in funding terms. However, there is some evidence that disputes about means in the NHS act as surrogates for disputes about ends since explicit disputes about the latter would be seen as illegitimate in a formally hierarchical Government agency (Elcock and Haywood, 1980 pp.49-50). A system of integrated planning and resource allocation, followed up by monitoring procedures with financial sanctions would inevitably bring into prominence conflicts over ends since there would be less scope for decentralised authorities to accept, resist or defer pressures to reorder their priorities. Although conflict avoidance is usually seen by managers of bureaucracies as a virtue, in this case, conflict would have the benefit of highlighting the key policy choices facing the NHS rather than permitting them to be fudged through the inertia of largely autonomous local health authorities. On the other hand, by making difficult policy choices explicit, the system could make the politicians' and policy-makers' lives more hazardous.

In the early part of this Chapter, Doreen Irving (Butts et al, 1981) showed how the organisation and functional divisions within the DHSS in the 1970s, particularly the bias towards individual client groups and muddled relations with the NHS, contributed to the de facto separation of planning from resource allocation. There have been considerable changes within DHSS since then to overcome a number of the problems to which she refers, culminating most recently in the establishment of an NHS Supervisory Board to look strategically at health policy and NHS objectives, in association with an NHS Management Board to provide a general management function at top level in the DHSS on behalf of the Secretary of State. Although it is still not clear exactly how the Management Board will relate to health authorities and whether it will perform a central management function for the NHS itself, it has the potential to do so (Halpern, 1985). The Management Board would then be able to provide some central direction to the NHS, and Regions would be accountable to the Board for attaining their objectives. Presumably such a system would make it possible to consider the inter-relationship of plans and resource allocation in a way which was not easy previously.

CHAPTER EIGHT

CONCLUSIONS

INTRODUCTION

This final Chapter aims to pull together the main conclusions of the literature review and link them to future directions for policy and research. A natural starting point is consideration of the issues identified in the terms of reference of the review of national RAWP by the NHS Management Board of DHSS which took place in 1986 (DHSS, 1986a). Of central concern to the review were questions of measuring morbidity and social deprivation. These were explicitly cited in the terms of reference, mentioned directly as two of the five aspects of particular interest and often taken to be implied in a third (inner cities). The two other aspects were teaching of medical students and accounting for cross-boundary flows. This Chapter discusses each of these issues. Although discussion of teaching does not draw directly on the literature reviewed here, it is included as it illustrates advantages of the integration of planning and resource allocation, which was a main theme of the previous Chapter ('RAWP and Planning'). The issues matter most not so much in the allocation of revenue to RHAs -- the concern of the DHSS RAWP review -- but in the process of sub-Regional resource allocation. This chapter therefore concentrates on sub-Regional issues. The final section proposes the main lines of future research suggested from writing this book.

MEASURING MORBIDITY

Nothing that RAWP did provoked as much argument as its choice of standardised mortality ratios (SMRs) as the means of measuring relative morbidity (see Chapters Four and Five). However, subsequent experience, criticism and research, have shown that RAWP, in most respects possessed remarkable soundness of judgement in its choice of information, boldness in conception, and grasp of the underlying objective and how in practice this might best be achieved. RAWP's choice of SMRs illustrates these and sadly much of the criticism falls far short of recognising the role of SMRs and why they were chosen.

The Impact of SMRs

First, it would be a mistake to exaggerate the importance of SMRs in RHAs' targets: the impression given by some criticisms is that SMRs bear the whole burden of measuring relative need; but they are a proxy for morbidity after a Region's age/sex structure has been accounted for. The population component of RAWP targets is dominated by population size and age/sex structure. The SMR is an additional refinement.

Problems of Measuring Morbidity

The second misconception of critics is a failure to appreciate that the measurement of morbidity is inevitably controversial. This controversy is, for example, illustrated by disagreements over statistical tests as indicators of morbidity from surveys of communities in the debate about the "clinical iceberg" of morbidity (Bradwell, Carnalt and Whitehead, 1974) and in reviews of hospital bed use over whether people are sick enough to justify the use of a bed. There was no perfect measure "out there" which RAWP overlooked, nor has subsequent research produced such a measure. Furthermore, arguments over competing measures of morbidity are over surrogate measures and direct measures rarely exist to enable the argument to be resolved (Mays, 1986).

Distinguishing Between Need and Demand

The third misconception, which characterises later rather than earlier criticism of the use of SMRs, is a failure to recognise that RAWP sought measures of need and not demand. Thus demonstrating that other measures are more successful than SMRs in "explaining" (in statistical models) variations in the use of services is irrelevant to RAWP's purpose. RAWP emphasised that it sought measures which were independent of supply, and analyses before and after the RAWP report show how supply dominates variables which explain variation in the uptake of services.

Measuring Relative Need Between Health Authorities

Many early critics of the choice of SMRs recognised the vital distinction between attempting to explain variations in satisfied demand (i.e. use) and measuring need. But they did not always appreciate that RAWP's requirement was not for measures of the absolute prevalence of all morbidity, but for indicators of relative morbidity between health authorities which they would be expected to treat. Forster's much cited paper (Forster, 1977), nicely illustrates this important distinction. SMRs were not closely correlated with those minor illnesses which were unlikely to place burdens on health authorities but were correlated with those which were. Forster and others failed to distinguish between these different types of diseases, and drew the wrong conclusion from such analyses: this work may be seen as strengthening the case for the choice of SMRs; they saw this work as evidence for their rejection.

Others have argued that the focus on mortality has meant the neglect of conditions which require health authority services but do not lead to death (Radical Statistics Health Group, 1977; Geary, 1977; Walker, 1978; Goldacre and Harris, 1980). But for RAWP's purpose what matters is whether there is geographic variation in these conditions. And again on these grounds the choice of SMRs seems to be vindicated: those conditions the incidence of which is likely to vary between health authorities tend to result in death; and those conditions which do not result in death tend to exhibit variations in incidence only between small areas (Bennett and Holland, 1977).

The Criticisms Summarised

The value of the above criticisms of SMRs is that they have enabled an appreciation to be made of what SMRs are and are not supposed to do. Such clarity does not always emerge from the necessarily terse account underlying their choice in the RAWP report. Furthermore we now have the advantages of hindsight in taking our position on this intensely debated topic. Criticisms remain over points of detail: such as the form in which mortality statistics should be aggregated (Palmer, West, Patrick and Glynn, 1979; Barr and Logan, 1977). RAWP chose mortality data because they are the most direct measure of morbidity, independent of supply, reliable and routinely available by age, sex, and diagnosis. No other measure of need has been proposed which is superior to mortality data on these criteria (Ashley and McLachlan, 1985). This does not mean that there is no scope for improvement, but this requires investment in measures of morbidity which are independent of supply. So far the NHS has failed to undertake such vital work, but this is the only way in which progress can be made from the position that RAWP reached in 1976.

There are further criticisms of RAWP's choice of SMRs which argue for a shift in RAWP's interpretation of its terms of reference. Indeed, over time, much of the criticism has shifted from disputing the adequacy of RAWP's proposed methods of achieving its underlying objective, to argue, implicitly or explicitly, that this objective be redefined. The greatest interest has been in redefining RAWP's "morbidity definition" of need to include social deprivation.

MEASURING SOCIAL DEPRIVATION

The measurement of "need" generates interest and debate because of problems of definition. Argument over RAWP's use of SMRs to measure need has been fruitful in clarifying how need is defined for RAWP's purposes. But no sooner has that argument run its course than a new one emerges. Although all measures of "morbidity" and "social deprivation" are strongly correlated, the choice of variable to use in the RAWP formula can have a marked impact on an authority's target. This means that an authority can choose to define social deprivation in terms of the variables which show that it "needs" most resources. One of the concerns about proposals to change the RAWP formula is that the fairness and objectivity of RAWP may be modified, with variables being added on grounds of political expediency in ways analogous to those of the rate support grant calculations (NAHA, 1986).

The discussion of social deprivation and RAWP tends to be confusing. This is because there are at least three arguments commonly used to justify incorporating social deprivation in RAWP target calculations. These are:

1. Social deprivation leads to a higher level of morbidity than indicated by mortality rates.

2. Social deprivation results in higher demands for and poorer access to services for any given level of morbidity.

3. The quality of primary care is poorer in deprived areas leading to a greater demand for hospital and community health services.

There is little evidence which enables the first argument to be quantified, and the third argument, though important, is not about social deprivation as such. Thus the core argument is the second: the extent, for example, that social deprivation results in longer hospital stays or the extent to which essential services (eg. prevention) are underused in deprived areas because of problems of access (Fox, 1978; Woods, 1982). But even the second argument does not point to an automatic adjustment to health authority targets to compensate for social deprivation in the community. It may indeed be the case that some people have to stay in hospital because of grossly inadequate housing, but it is odd to see the necessary response as a permanent adjustment in hospital finances rather than directly remedying inadequate housing. Furthermore, on a simple level of correlation, studies show that SMRs and measures of social deprivation are highly associated at District level. It appears that the adverse conditions experienced by socially deprived people are reflected in their mortality rates.

RHAs' responses to the problems of accounting for morbidity and social deprivation in sub-Regional RAWP are misguided in two respects. First, they seek to measure both morbidity and social deprivation with one indicator that derives weights from the existing use of services (North East Thames Regional Health Authority, 1983a and 1983b; North West Thames Regional Health Authority, undated). RAWP sought a measure of need independent of service use, knowing that use mainly reflects supply, and that there is no better indicator of morbidity than mortality. Thus

RHAs would be better advised to seek to measure the extra burden of social deprivation beyond relative morbidity as indicated by mortality data. Second, work ought not to be directed at some comprehensive indicator which may be a product of the "ecological fallacy". Populations as defined by DHAs include a mix of people, and it may be that the heavier use of services identified and rewarded by these indicators is not because of the deprived individuals, but because of others who are not "deprived" but skilled at placing their demands on health authorities. It is thus important to be specific about which particular aspects of social deprivation are relevant to the need for health services and how services ought to be developed to respond. However, studies of how "social deprivation" affects the "need" for health services, typically avoid being specific in these ways.

The approach to seeking "social deprivation" weights in RAWP reinforces the long-running fallacy that spending more on health services in deprived areas is an appropriate response to the needs of those who are socially deprived. For over a hundred years, Britain has provided a rich diet of health services in some of its most deprived areas. Yet, far less attention has been given to tackling the underlying causes of the problems faced by people in those areas.

INNER CITIES

Inner cities are not the only places where social deprivation occurs, although inner city deprivation has characteristics which make it easy to identify, particulary visually (through photographs and television). Two points seem to matter as regards cities. One, mentioned above, is the quality of primary care. The second is the effect of London on pay and conditions necessary to attract staff. Neither of these is straightforward to identify and remedy.

Analyses of spending on General Medical Services (GMS) - provided by GPs - shows that GMS spending is weakly correlated with the distribution of resources to health authorities (Bevan and Charlton, 1986). However, high spending by GPs may occur for reasons quite unconnected with the volume of services delivered: there are ways of organising practices which generate large fixed payments from Family Practitioner Committees (London Health Planning Consortium, 1981). Thus it is necessary to get behind the payments to see what kind of services are delivered in cities. On this point there is no consistent picture: problems have been identified in London but not in Manchester (Wood, 1983; Wilkin, Metcalfe, Hallam, Cooke and Hodgkin, 1984). Inner cities only provide a special case of the general problem of how resources allocated to health authorities can be constructively related to payments made to GMS. Both RAWP and the Advisory Group on Resource Allocation (AGRA) (DHSS, 1980b), were concerned about this failure. Nothing has been done, however, to address it, and indeed in England, the 1982 reorganisation added a further obstacle to closer integration of these two services by giving FPCs independence from DHAs and creating them as authorities in their own right.

The second problem is that of geographical variations in pay. DHSS (but not all RHAs) makes allowance in addition to "London weighting" on pay, for "London market costs" based on analyses done some years ago of the extra labour market costs in London (Weeden, 1980). In addition to the need to bring this analysis up to date, there is a problem yet to be satisfactorily resolved: the allowance is based solely on staff for whom the NHS is in competition with other employers and excludes, nurses, doctors, etc.. This is a reasonable first approximation to studying labour market cost variations, but it overlooks the conditions of and competition for professional staff between health authorities within the NHS. For example, it seems plausible that London authorities may have to provide more accommodation for nurses than other authorities to attract and retain staff, given the relative costs of housing in London and elsewhere. This problem has yet to be satisfactorily analysed.

ACCOUNTING FOR CROSS BOUNDARY FLOWS

Adequacy of RAWP Methods in Accounting for Flows

The typical arguments about cross-boundary flows are that patients who are referred for treatment across boundaries and to teaching hospitals are more complex than patients treated in the District where they live; but, that the adjustments made for cross-boundary flows are based on national average costs by specialty which fail to give adequate compensation for the more complex case-mix of cross-boundary flow patients (Royal Commission on the National Health Service, 1978b; Radical Statistics Health Group, 1977). The available evidence suggests, however, that current methods are adequate in terms of adjustments to targets. Regional targets have been shown to be largely insensitive to these adjustments (DHSS, 1980b). Sub-Regionally, such research as there has been into the case-mix of flows, has shown RAWP methods to be fair (Akehurst and Johnson, 1980). Furthermore, RHAs typically make special provision for high-cost Regional (or multi-District) specialties, and it is reasonable to suppose that other cases are adequately compensated for by average costs (DHSS, 1980b).

Unfortunately, the adequacy of current methods of accounting for costs of residents of one authority treated in another does not mean that the methods currently used are, or will continue to be, satisfactory. Problems are likely to arise from better information as this will make clear the incentive effects of the methods which are used (NHS/DHSS Steering Group on Health Services Information, 1984a and 1984b).

Incentive Effects of RAWP Methods

Allowance is made in targets for flows of inpatients but not dayand outpatients. As Regions' allocations come closer to targets, this will increasingly generate incentives not to use dayand outpatient care, despite these commonly being economical alternatives to inpatient care. The introduction of the Korner information systems might be used to record cross-boundary flows of dayand outpatients. This would enable these flows to be included in RAWP and eliminate the undesirable incentives of current methods.

At present, hospitals typically only know the average costs per inpatient case and only exceptionally, the costs of the different types of cases that they treat. Even with this limited knowledge, sub-Regional RAWP (based on the Net Flow method of national RAWP) generates (unintended) incentives because it uses two different concepts of fairness. The first concept is that of fair shares of revenue by population. This is intended to dominate the composition of targets and does so for RHAs, but not for many inner city DHAs. The second concept of fairness is that an authority ought to be adequately reimbursed for the patients it treats who live in other authorities. Authorities which have residents using more (or less) than their fair share will have in their targets sums which are correspondingly less (or more) than the costs of their residents' current use of services. This means authorities will be allowed less (or more) than national average costs for treating their own residents. But authorities are allowed average costs in their targets for treating residents of other authorities. Hence financial incentives exist to discriminate between residents and non-residents (Bevan and Brazier, 1985a and 1985b). These incentives are neither intuitive nor benign, since they encourage over-target DHAs to treat residents of neighbouring DHAs as inpatients as often as possible and their own residents as economically as possible. If each DHA were to do this then none would have resources left (after deductions for their own residents treated in other DHAs) to treat their own residents (Bevan and Brazier, 1986).

Modifying RAWP Methods

Although methods other than the Net Flow Method of RAWP have been proposed for estimating catchment populations, Regional targets are likely to be robust to choice of methods. However, the Treatment Intensity method recommended by the Acute Services Working Group of the Joint Group on Performance Indicators (DHSS, 1984b) is difficult to understand, less stable than the Net Flow method, and vulnerable to manipulation by reporting flow statistics (Beech, Craig and Bevan, 1987; Bevan, 1986; Bevan and Ingram, 1986).

When DHAs know costs of cases in greater detail than they do now, incentive effects will be obvious, and there will be pressure for refinements in cost adjustments for treating residents of other DHAs. This will inevitably lead to problems. A DHA may know that it has spent much more than the standard costs in treating residents of other DHAs, yet the NHS can hardly afford to respond by introducing a method which reimburses DHAs for the full costs of cases treated: even the USA can no longer afford to do this (Iglehart, 1982). Thus the prospects are for contested negotiations over "reasonable" costs for cross-boundary flows.

Cross-charging

There is already interest in moving towards a system of cross-charging whereby DHAs negotiate contracts with each other on a competitive basis. It is sometimes argued that this market-based approach will lead to higher quality care at lower cost, but there are deficiencies in the basic information necessary for knowing whether these benefits are or are not being secured. Evaluating the success of cross-charging requires far superior measures of costs, case-mix, and quality than will be routinely available even when the teething troubles of the Korner recommendations on NHS information systems have been overcome. Thus the alleged benefits of cross-charging can only rest on faith that such changes will bring them about (Brazier, 1986).

The interest in cross-charging may be seen as seizing on one aspect of Enthoven's recent proposals for transforming DHAs into Health Maintenance Organisations (HMOs) in which DHAs would receive the residential component of their RAWP targets and then decide the most efficient way of providing services for their residents on a competitive basis. Competition could be between: services on their own premises from their own employees or from the private sector; services from other DHAs; or services from private hospitals (Enthoven, 1985a). Enthoven's exposition of his ideas was lucid, brief and highlighted important changes necessary for his proposals to be implemented successfully. He, however, omitted to draw attention to the requirements for improved information which cannot be dismissed as trivial or merely technical - consider the largely unresolved problems of measuring quality of care! But there was one vital change to the NHS which he recognised as fundamental to securing the full realisation of the management culture he believed to be necessary for his ideas to work, and that was the ending of free choice of physician. In his scheme, GPs would be under the control of DHAs and lose their freedom to refer patients to any hospital physician. Such changes are inescapable if services for DHA residents are to be meaningfully negotiated. Whereas in Scotland GPs are closely administratively integrated with Health Boards, in England they are independent and thus what Enthoven has suggested would require major and unwelcome changes for GPs.

Enthoven has emphasised that the crucial change enabling US health care costs to be contained, in what he called the transformation 'from guild to market',is the ending of free choice of physician (Enthoven, 1985b). This enables choice to be restricted to physicians who accept responsibility for rationing resources. Analysis of the success of HMOs in containing costs shows that this is in the main due to reductions in inpatient referral rates (Manning et al, 1984). Thus cross-charging under cost containment by cash limits requires much more explicit control over inpatient referrals and must end the current free choice of hospital by patients, GPs and hospital doctors. This implies not only restrictions in where referrals can be made, but also limits on the volume of total referrals. Perhaps the most important point to emerge from analysing the incentive effects of sub-Regional RAWP is that the financial problems of, for example, London's teaching hospitals are not due to inadequate compensation for treating residents of other DHAs, but caused by the relatively excessive use of inpatient services by their residents both within and outside their DHA (Bevan and Brazier, 1985b). Thus, the application of cross-charging to these DHAs on the basis of an equitable distribution of revenue would require reductions in their residents' use of services.

FINANCING THE SERVICE COSTS OF MEDICAL STUDENT TRAINING

Before DHSS applies the RAWP formula to decide how to allocate revenue to RHAs, monies are set aside ("top-sliced") for selected purposes from the total revenue allocation to English authorities. The most significant purpose, in terms of the scale of money reserved for it, is for the medical Service Increment for Teaching (SIFT), which is intended solely to cover the extra service costs incurred by the NHS in the clinical training of medical students (DHSS, 1976c). This totalled £226m in 1985-86, and RHAs received £25,000 for each student being trained (DHSS, 1985b). Whether SIFT is or is not adequate for its designated purpose has been disputed since it was first proposed. The process of deriving the medical SIFT rate as the basis for allocating SIFT to health authorities is a source of confusion and controversy. RAWP bears the blame for this as it set the terms and tone of the ensuing debate. RAWP's grasp of other issues was so secure that its proposals have proved adequate well beyond the objective of its deliberations (setting a basis for equalising allocations to RHAs largely through growth over a ten year period). In contrast, its exposition of the derivation of SIFT was unclear (and led to the commonly expressed view that teaching hospitals only get 75% of what they are fairly entitled to); and the concepts underlying its derivation are incompatible with how RHAs are required to distribute revenue to DHAs. Although the derivation and allocation of SIFT are unsound and incoherent (Bevan, 1982b), RAWP's proposals were adequate for deciding RHA allocations through growth. However, problems arise when SIFT is used alongside RAWP to decide reductions in revenue allocations to DHAs.

RAWP methods have already been shown to use two principles of financing health services: the residential component of targets is based on finance by capitation; compensation for cross-boundary flows is based on finance by activity. This illustrates the problem of aiming to finance services by capitation where it is difficult to define the population to be served. Under these circumstances the natural recourse is to finance by activity. Although the provision of SIFT is quite obviously another adjustment to the target in terms of finance by activity, its incompatibility with the supposedly main principle of finance by capitation has hardly been noticed. This incompatibility constitutes one of the fundamental flaws in the derivation of SIFT.

In estimating the medical SIFT rate per student the aim was to find out how much extra ought to be allocated to teaching hospitals beyond the estimated costs of their service activities at the level of the "45 hospitals' sample formula". This formula was based on the costs of the most modern hospitals in England and Wales and was the basis of the generous funding of the Revenue Consequences of Capital Schemes (RCCS) - a DHSS practice that ended following the introduction of RAWP methods. This cost level was chosen because it was assumed that the unit costs of teaching hospitals ought to be at the level of the most modern hospitals. The costing base was crude (and the later revision of the SIFT rate by AGRA took only approximate account of teaching hospitals' case-mix) (Bevan, 1982b). For each medical school, its 'teaching hospitals' were identified and 'excess costs' derived, defined as the difference between actual expenditures (less London Weighting where relevant) and the 'baseline service costs'. Difficulties were identified with the method because of the wide range of 'excess costs per student' by medical school, and the problem of deciding how to use these data to derive a fair allowance for SIFT.

After SIFT had been used for a number of years, DHSS commissioned a study from Professor Perrin on the feasibility of estimating the costs of clinical training of medical students by using accounting methods, since this was seen to be the main problem with the process of estimating SIFT (Perrin and Magee, 1982). Perrin and Magee argued, however, that the first priority in understanding why teaching hospitals were more expensive than other hospitals, was to examine the costs of their case-mix. This was their main 'product' and ought to be more adequately costed than in the methods used by RAWP and AGRA to derive estimates of SIFT. Understanding the costs of their main activity was likely to be more rewarding than seeking to separate out the costs of clinical teaching from the other jointly-produced outputs of teaching hospitals. This was because there is massive overlap in the people employed on routine and specialised care, teaching (of medical students and other staff), and research (Culyer and Drummond, 1978). The corollary of this argument is that where there are problems in financing teaching hospitals, the first point to examine is how their cases are financed rather than whether SIFT is or is not adequate for the extra costs of clinical teaching of medical students.

DHSS Performance Indicators for 1983-84 (DHSS, 1985a) show teaching hospitals' actual inpatient expenditures to be close to the expected costs of their inpatient cases at national average costs with allowances for teaching (and London where relevant). A case study of St Thomas' showed that the allowances made by RAWP methods and DHSS Performance Indicators for the total costs of London and teaching were similar, but the target allowances for inpatient cases (even after allowing for Regional specialties) were much less than the national average costs of inpatient cases by specialty (Bevan and Brazier, 1985a and 1985b). This suggests that if teaching hospitals were funded at national average costs for the cases they treat, together with SIFT, they would not be in financial difficulties. Furthermore, if they were funded on the basis of the derivation of SIFT, at the more generous level for the "45 hospital sample" costs, with due allowance for their more complex case-mix, some at least would receive increased allocations.

The fundamental point is that policy since RAWP has been to finance hospitals not by their activity but by an equitable distribution of revenue based on capitation. SIFT is allocated to protect the extra costs arising from the training of medical students, but derived from methods which assumed a generous cost estimate for the cases teaching hospitals treat. The problem may be illustrated, quite simply. Consider a teaching hospital with an annual intake of 100 medical students. The guidance of the University Grants Committee (UGC) is that these students require 200 beds in general medicine and general surgery. Suppose the costs of clinical training of the students in these specialties are £4m, the service costs amount to £20m, and finance by capitation through RAWP gives target funding of £10m for 100 beds. Then if SIFT fully covers the costs of clinical training, the hospital may expect eventual funding of £14m against its total costs of £24m. Even if the SIFT allowance were quite correct, the hospital operating efficiently, and its case-mix adequately accounted for, it would still have a financial problem. This is because there is a prior issue to be resolved which lay outside RAWP's remit, namely, how to reconcile an equitable distribution of resources to populations with those required for training medical students.

Confusion over SIFT includes other aspects of its derivation. The student rate is set at 75% of the 'median excess costs per student', and this is why it is commonly and erroneously believed that teaching hospitals are deprived of 25% of their entitlement. The choice of the 75% figure is justified by reference to the "York Study" (Culyer, Wiseman, Drummond and West, 1978). The study estimated the higher costs incurred by teaching hospitals in the clinical training of medical students on a quite different basis from RAWP and AGRA. Different data were used (different samples of teaching and non-teaching hospitals with data from different years) and different methods (the "York Study" used an econometric model). The study is thus largely irrelevant to the decision by RAWP (and AGRA) about the proportion of the estimated excess costs per student which should be used to set the SIFT rate (Bevan, 1982b). RAWP wanted to set SIFT at a rate that erred on the side of generosity, but did not err too much! The full median cost was judged to be too high; 50% presumably judged too low: and 75% felt to be about right! It appears that it was this judgement which underlay the choice of 75% and the York result was cited in support of that judgement rather than as a direct cause of it. Thus the adequacy or otherwise of SIFT cannot be determined by the way it was derived. If, however, a teaching hospital is given the choice of either medical students, their extra costs, and the corresponding SIFT; or no students, no extra costs and no SIFT, the hospital would almost certainly be better off with the former than the latter.

In presenting its allowance for SIFT, RAWP drew attention to a conflict between "excellence" and equity, and thus gave its authority to a common view that the financial problems of teaching hospitals caused by RAWP's methods are due to this conflict. RAWP was hardly likely to have been conscious of the implications of these remarks, particularly as its methods and subsequent developments have meant that much of the "excellence" of teaching hospitals has been specially protected. RAWP itself intended SIFT to be overgenerous for the teaching of medical students, and this appears to be so. In addition, since RAWP reported, special arrangements have been made for the high cost Regional Specialties commonly provided by teaching hospitals. Given these arrangements, teaching hospitals are reasonably compensated by the use of estimated national average costs by specialty for the remaining inpatients they treat in general acute specialties who live outside their DHAs. The financial problems of teaching hospitals appear to arise because the residents of the DHAs in which the hospitals are situated make heavier use of inpatient services than can be afforded by an equitable distribution of the current total available to RHAs.

SUBREGIONAL RESOURCE ALLOCATION

Sub-Regional RAWP

The use of RAWP as a means of deciding sub-Regional resource allocation rests on three assumptions: that the formula is a good indicator of an equitable distribution of revenue; that the incentives of its application are appropriate; and that responsibility for the attainment of its underlying objectives can sensibly be devolved to DHAs. The focus of attention of the literature has been on the first of these assumptions. The criticisms of the past decade have mainly shown the formula to be a robust and reliable indicator of a fair distribution of total resources to health authorities' populations for RAWP's purposes. Studies have shown that: there is no measure of relative morbidity independent of supply superior to mortality; it is doubtful if the assessment of relative morbidity is improved by the addition of an allowance for social deprivation; the cross-boundary flow adjustments for acute inpatients are adequate; and medical SIFT probably errs on the side of generosity for the costs of clinical training of medical students. Thus as a means of indicating relative entitlement to total resources, RAWP targets are likely to be reliable for most authorities, and possibly overgenerous for teaching authorities.

The problems of accounting for cross-boundary flows for Regional and general acute services arise not so much from the level of reimbursement for these activities, as from the incentive effects that follow when RHAs use RAWP methods and devolve responsibility for achieving target allocations to DHAs. The adjustments for cross-boundary flows do not matter where they are relatively small in proportion to the capitation-based element, that is for RHAs and rural, non-teaching DHAs. The adjustments undermine the basis of RAWP when they dominate targets of inner-city, teaching DHAs. The incentive effects of the protection of Regional Specialties are obvious: there is often controversy over the volume of cases RHAs are prepared to finance. For other cross-boundary flows, the incentives are latent, but would be potentially more devastating if they were followed. Inner city teaching DHAs have a further adjustment to the capitation element of targets in the form of SIFT which effectively makes them responsible for reconciling bed requirements for teaching medical students with an equitable distribution of services. They are poorly placed to do this.

Any system of redistribution without growth will be highly unpopular with those who face cuts. Much of the criticism of RAWP is simply because of this and would lase were redistribution to be financed by growth, which was how RAWP saw its methods being applied. Methods of redistribution without growth must be soundly based where cuts are necessary. Unfortunately the application of RAWP is weakest in determining allocations precisely where targets show that substantial cuts in services have to be made to finance redistribution. Inner city, teaching DHAs are important not only because of the complex range of services and needs they meet, but also because, given little or no growth in the total budget for health authorities, these authorities are the "bank" to finance redistribution.

One of the difficulties in making sense of RAWP is that its application has quite different meanings to different authorities: for RHAs it is sound and implies gradual change; for rural, DHAs outside cities and without major teaching responsibilities, it is sound and promises real growth; for inner city, teaching DHAs it is unsound and requires cuts. RAWP seems to be perfectly reasonable to authorities other than inner city, teaching DHAs. Yet, the criticisms expressed by these inner city DHAs are rarely based on a full understanding of why RAWP is unsound as applied to them. This is most clearly illustrated in the typical District response to the need to reduce expenditure. Priority tends to be given to local residents and cuts made in services for others. However, the incentives of sub-Regional RAWP are quite the opposite. Another example is the familiar argument that SIFT is inadequate, whereas the problem is not so much with funding the extra costs of clinical training but with maintaining the services necessary to support that training.

Health Authorities as Trading Organisations

Health Authorities typically see their financial allocations as unaffected by their activities. This would be the case if all their revenue were decided by their resident population. This would be the equivalent of HMOs with membership decided by DHA of residence as proposed by Enthoven (1985a). But sub-Regional RAWP means that targets and hence future allocations, are affected by the numbers of: cases treated in Regional Specialties; residents of other DHAs treated as inpatients; DHA residents treated as inpatients in other DHAs; and medical students trained (Bevan, 1986). These rules, together with lags in adjustments to targets, and indirect links between targets and allocations, result in an odd set of "terms of trade". In contrast, cross-charging is attractive because its rules are simple and direct and insist that DHAs control the inpatient referrals of their residents by restricting choice and limiting volume. For inner city, teaching DHAs, this implies reducing the volume of their residents' admissions but it is not at all clear as to how this should be achieved in the current NHS. The difficulty is that evidence consistently shows that hospital beds are filled largely by people who lived close to them. Although teaching hospitals in cities treat as inpatients many non-DHA residents (and in London, many from other RHAs), this is often evidence of the arbitrary nature of DHA and RHA boundaries, rather than of large numbers of referrals over long distances. If cross-charging as a means of redistribution without growth is not to mean cuts in beds in inner city teaching DHAs, then it implies altering bed use in hospitals away from those who live locally (regardless of whether they live in the same DHA or RHA) towards those living in remote places. Where this alteration is not achieved, bed cuts are likely to be necessary which in turn would raise the problem of ensuring that teaching requirements match the ensuing distribution of beds.

Cross-charging is one way of altering sub-Regional RAWP by putting the adjustments for activity on a more straightforward basis. But this raises problems of reconciling the incentives of payment by activity (which are to increase the volume) with a cash limit allocated mainly on the principle of capitation. Furthermore, cross-charging raises all the problems discussed in the USA of attempting to set fair rates of reimbursement for case-mix groups. For the USA, fixing rates of reimbursement prospectively is a natural step in attempting to contain costs given that finance is by charges for services delivered. The NHS has another model available for distributing finance: namely, by planning hospitals in relation to populations and financing them for the likely costs of their services. Although this approach has become unfashionable, it is worth examining more closely some of the reasons for this, and discussing its future potential.

Regional Strategic Management

The 1962 Hospital Plan made logical sense: equalisation of resources to populations was to be achieved primarily through the distribution of capital, and revenue would follow when the facilities existed to make good use of it (Ministry of Health, 1962). As the process based on the Plan developed, it neglected two vital aspects which understandably brought the process into disrepute. First, the Plan applied only to Regional Hospital Boards (RHBs) and excluded teaching hospitals. Although the Plan's objective was greater equity, the massive rebuilding programme of London's teaching hospitals, agreed outside the Plan, meant that inequities were worsened through the building of new hospitals (Bennett and Holland, 1977). The administrative separation of teaching from other hospitals would not have undermined the achievement of greater equity without a second failure: the lack of adequate monitoring of planned developments and their revenue consequences. Indeed, generous granting of the Revenue Consequences of Capital Schemes (RCCS) meant that, as RAWP observed, bids for capital became means of boosting revenue rather than directing scarce resources to the future alleviation of inequality.

In arguing for strategic management of resources whereby inequality is remedied by relating revenue to the capacity to make good use of it, it is helpful to point to ways in which this approach can avoid the errors of the process based on the 1962 Hospital Plan. Two important errors have been rectified: most teaching hospitals are now administered by RHAs and DHAs and funding of RCCS has been abandoned by DHSS. Although RHAs vary in how they fund the running costs of new hospitals, if RCCS is granted, it is commonly tied in with redistribution of revenue as indicated by RAWP targets. Thus RAWP targets provide a means of monitoring the distribution of resources, and provide an approximate check against the concentration of hospital building in particular areas. Nevertheless, there is value in producing more sensitive indicators to monitor RHAs' strategic intentions, to ensure, for example, that these make sense across RHA boundaries.

Strategic management is an alternative to sub-Regional RAWP and is a practical means of financing by capitation at sub-Regional level (Bevan, Beech and Craig, 1985). The objective is to distribute hospital capacity and revenue in relation to the relative need of populations (Bevan, 1986). Experience shows that people tend to use the most convenient hospital. Thus equalising accessibility to capacity will lead to equitable use of services. Need can be estimated by following the

RAWP method of weighting populations by age, sex and SMRs and any other better morbidity measures if they become available. However, in contrast to RAWP and cross-charging, health authority boundaries are disregarded in a strategic view of the redistribution of acute services.

Strategic management, unlike RAWP and cross-charging, would focus on the difficult task of managing change from a Regional perspective, because RHAs unlike DHAs can make coherent sense of how a Region's acute services ought to be distributed. This means, for example, checking that increases in revenue are tied to the capacity to make good use of it; examining the various flows of monies necessary to finance proposed commitments in acute services (such as commissioning new hospitals) and "priority services" (such as providing community-based care) to see that they are not vulnerable to future uncertainties (such as underfunding of pay awards). It is paradoxical that this approach should be seen as somehow different from sub-Regional RAWP, because, apart from refining formulae, RHAs' main role in the use of targets to decide DHA allocations lies in setting the pace of change. If this is to be done in other than a mechanical manner, then it requires the kind of assessments involved in strategic management. Seen in this way it seems odd for a RHA to use a strategy to make these assessments and then revert to sub-Regional RAWP as the means of deciding future allocations. But, presumably this is what happens in RHAs where strategic planning and resource allocation are imperfectly coordinated.

In practice, Regional strategic management is none other than actively managing the changes indicated by sub-Regional RAWP by adopting a regional perspective. This brings three immediate advantages for resolving the problems of inner city, teaching DHAs. First, equity between Districts is a concept which RHA members can make sense of, whereas DHA members owe their primary allegiance to their residents and staff. DHA comparisons make abundantly clear the scale of unequal use of services and where, given a fixed budget, cuts and increases ought to take place. DHAs find it difficult to accept that their residents are making an excessive use of services, because, as RAWP recognised, demand increases beyond available supply. Thus to DHA members, services always appear to be inadequate for their residents. To ask DHAs to implement policies to promote equity through RAWP results in nonsenses: either they ignore what RAWP requires and aim to preserve services for their residents, which risks reductions in targets and the need for more cuts; or they follow the implicit financial incentives of RAWP with farcical results, ending up bankrupting each other by trying to admit as many non-residents as possible. This illustrates the second difficulty facing DHA members and the second advantage of Regional strategic management: even if DHAs wanted to do so, how can they make their residents' use of services more equitable, given the extent of cross-boundary flows? This would not be a problem under strategic management which ignores these boundaries for acute hospital services. The third emerging difficulty for inner-city, teaching DHAs, which regional strategic management is better equipped to address is how to match an equitable distribution of services with teaching requirements. A Regional, if not a national, perspective seems to be essential for this. From a Regional perspective it is easier to assess service and teaching requirements for beds in the core specialties of general medicine and general surgery, the gap between them, and the various ways of reconciling the likely conflict. The policy issues to be resolved are over the number and distribution of medical students and how they are to be trained.

Regional strategic management clarifies implications of current policies and responsibilities for resolving the problems thus identified. This is at one and the same time a strength and weakness. Equalisation without growth entails significant reductions of inpatient beds in inner London and hospital closures. RHAs are well placed to make coherent sense of the implications of these policies, but spelling these out is unpopular and conflicts with traditions of local autonomy. The implementation of Regional strategic management will test government commitment to the pursuit of equity by demonstrating its costs. Without Ministerial backing for unpopular decisions, there is little point in seeking to make strategic sense of the problems facing London. This raises the keenly-debated topic of whether enough is spent in total on the NHS. We briefly explore this in suggesting an agenda for future research.

AN AGENDA FOR FUTURE RESEARCH

Although the review of the RAWP formula by the NHS Management Board is concerned with its application by DHSS to Regions, the serious problems arise in making sub-Regional allocations. Inequity is much greater sub-Regionally and achieving equity without growth implies major reductions in revenue for some DHAs, in particular, inner London, teaching DHAs. Sub-Regional RAWP is inadequate as a means of resolving these problems. The fashionable alternative of cross-charging whilst simplifying the "terms of trade" for health authorities, brings other major problems such as controlling the pattern of referrals to hospitals by independent GPs. Regional strategic management is not an easy option, as it will make the implications of the pursuit of sub-Regional equity without growth abundantly clear. This will lead to the question being asked as to whether or not government policy ought simply to be concerned with the achievement of equity, without any explicit consideration of the nature of the equity being sought. To begin to answer this fundamental question, it is essential for research to go beyond the position RAWP reached in 1976.

This book has argued that RAWP was correct in its hypothesis that the principal explanation for variations in the use of services (having taken account of age, sex and SMRs) is variations in access to supply. This, however, does not dispose of the matter. There is no evidence to show that people in hospital beds in London are not clinically in need of treatment (Beech, Challah and Ingram, 1987). There is a deeply felt belief that some people cannot get the treatment they need currently, even in the best-off DHAs facing RAWP cuts, and that the consequences of these cuts will be an inhumane practice of medicine. This belief may be at the root of the various arguments about international comparisons of NHS expenditure, lack of growth of the NHS, social deprivation and inadequate funding of SIFT. A line of inquiry we see as relevant to decisions about future funding of the NHS would be to investigate such questions as: how do differences in supply in different parts of the country affect referrals by GPs and decisions to admit by hospital doctors; and what impact do differing admission rates have on the health of populations?

In many ways RAWP's methods provide a useful pointer to further research and development of policies by health authorities. Four such have emerged from writing this book.

The first is to develop a constructive approach to measuring and coping with social deprivation. A working hypothesis, which remains to be tested, is that RAWP's age, sex and SMR weighting takes account of differences in relative morbidity, but not the extra burdens which health authorities have to cope with from operating in socially deprived areas. Analyses of current patterns of use are contaminated by supply and thus cannot provide satisfactory evidence of these burdens. Instead, the task is to identify the special provision merited by various characteristics of social deprivation, so that if extra resources were allocated for social deprivation they could be related to specific services.

The second direction is to refine RAWP's remarkably durable working hypothesis that SMRs are adequate proxies for morbidity. This will require specially designed surveys. As in the investigation of social deprivation, such surveys ought to be directed at conditions where health authorities are believed to be failing to match services to needs. There should be clear policies as to how the results of surveys will be used to alter the delivery of services.

The third direction is to develop skills in regional strategic management. At the time of going to press, the attempt of one RHA to use this process as the basis of resource allocation has run into problems (Hodges, 1986). It is difficult to relate resources to strategies which focus on precise forecasts of what is to be achieved at the end of the strategic period, because forecasts are invariably wrong. There is much written and talked about the vital importance of developing robust strategies to cope with future uncertainty, but this too is difficult in practice. What is needed here is an unusual combination of research and practice to show how this can be done by RHAs.

The final point on resource allocation concerns the finance of teaching hospitals: where RAWP failed to provide a firm basis for the future. This might seem a strange issue on which to focus, since most health authorities would regard it as relatively unimportant and special pleading by a privileged elite. But teaching DHAs are commonly at the centre of arguments over redistribution, and the service requirements of teaching are emerging as major potential obstacles to making sense of those arguments. The UGC recommendations of bed numbers for teaching are not inviolable. What is required is an examination of bed requirements of teaching and how they conflict with an equitable distribution of services (Holland, 1984 and 1986). When the scale of the conflict is known, options can be investigated for its resolution.

RAWP stands out as a signal success in public policy initiatives over the last twenty years, particularly when compared with other failed attempts to apply rational approaches in public policy. RAWP was preceded in the UK by the Roskill Commission's use of cost-benefit analysis to recommend a site for a third London airport which has had no impact on decisions by the Government (Bevan, 1975; Departments of the Environment and of Transport, undated); and in the USA by the abandonment of Plan-Program-Budgeting-System (PPBS) (Dennison, 1979; Wildavsky, 1974). RAWP was followed by the failure of the attempts to improve the distribution of the local authority Rate Support Grant which was closely analogous to RAWP in its objective (Gibson and Travers, 1985). Why was RAWP in contrast so successful? There are important lessons of policy implementation to be learned of far wider significance than the NHS. Chapter Two on the historical background to RAWP amounts to no more than a preliminary sketch. Resource allocation to health authorities was fundamentally altered by the RAWP report. Its underlying objective and chosen methods of measuring an appropriate distribution of resources are likely to be profoundly influential for the foreseeable future. It is therefore fitting that we should try better to understand the ingredients of a remarkable initiative.

REFERENCES

B. Abel-Smith (1978),   National Health Service: The First Thirty Years , HMSO, London.

B. Abel-Smith (1981),   'United Kingdom experience with sharing health resources between the Regions', in D.M.   Salter (ed)   Health Planning and Resource Allocation,   Wellington Clinical School of Medicine, Wellington, NZ, pp. 53-9.

R.M. Acheson (1978),   'The definition and identification of need for health care', Journal of Epidemiology and Community Health, 32, 10-15.

R.L. Akehurst and K.W. Johnson (1980), 'Cross-boundary flows of patients: the effect of adjusting sub-Regional target revenue allocations for case mix within the North Western RHA', Hospital and Health Services Review, 76: 10, 334-6.

D. Allen (1981),   'An analysis of the factors affecting the development of the 1962 Hospital Plan for England and Wales', Social Policy and Administration, 15, 3-18.

Anonymous (1975a),   'Painful redistribution', British Medical Journal, iv, 66-7.

Anonymous (1975b),   'Fair shares', Hospital and Health Services Review, 71: 12, 413-4.

Anonymous (1976a),   'The end of excellence?' British Medical Journal, ii, 779-80.

Anonymous (1976b),   'What a RAWP roar', British Medical Journal, ii, 1280.

Anonymous (1978),   'Time to rawp RAWP?' World Medicine, 1 November, 5.

Anonymous (1985),   'Wide variations in hospital waiting times and lists', British Medical Journal, 290, 577-8.

J.R. Ashford, K.L.O. Read and V.C. Riley (1973), 'An analysis of variations in perinatal mortality amongst local authorities in England and Wales', International Journal of Epidemiology, 2, 31 - 46.

J. Ashley and G. McLachlan (eds) (1985), Mortal or Morbid? A Diagnosis of the Morbidity Factor. Report of a NPHT Working Party, NPHT Occasional Hundred, no.10, Nuffield Provincial Hospitals Trust, London.

F. Avery-Jones (1976), 'The London Hospitals' scene', British Medical Journal, ii, 1046-9.

F. Avery-Jones (1978), 'The RAWP of London', World Medicine, 1 November, 19-22.

F. Avery-Jones (1979), 'RAWP, The Royal Commission and the "inner cities"', Lancet, ii, 372-374.

M.R. Baker and E.E.M. Kernohan (1985), Ethnic Minorities and the Cost of Care in the Community, Paper to 29th Annual Scientific Meeting of the Society for Social Medicine, 11-13 September 1985, University of Bradford, Clinical Epidemiology Research Unit, Bradford, unpublished.

R. Balarajan (1986), 'On the state of health in inner London', British Medical Journal, 292, 911-4.

A. Barr and R.F.L. Logan (1977), 'Policy alternatives for resource allocation', Lancet, i, 994-6.

R. Beech, M. Craig and G. Bevan (1987), ' Estimating catchment populations: implications for target allocations', Hospital and Health Services Review, in press.

R. Beech, S. Challah and R.H. Ingram (1987), 'The impact of cuts in acute beds on patient services', British Medical Journal, in press.

A.E. Bennett and W.W. Holland (1977), 'Rational planning or muddling through? Resource allocation in the NHS,' Lancet, i, 464-6.

R.L. Berg (ed) (1973), Health Status Indexes, Hospital Research and Education Trust, Chicago.

R.G. Bevan (1975), 'Operational Research and the pluralist frame of reference', Omega, 3:6, 699-708.

G. Bevan (1982a), 'Using gravity to put muscle into RAWP', The Health Services, 12 November, 10.

R.G. Bevan (1982b), A Critique of the Medical Service Increment for Teaching (SIFT), Warwick Papers in Industry, Business and Administration, No.6., University of Warwick, Centre for Research in Industry, Business and Administration, School of Industrial and Business Studies, Coventry.

R.G. Bevan (1984), 'Organising the finance of hospitals by simulated markets', Fiscal studies, 5, 44-62.

R.G. Bevan (1985), Is Variation in Expenditure per Head of English FPCs on General Medical Services in 1980-81 Due to Variation in Composition of FPCs' Accounts? Department of Community Medicine, United Medical and Dental Schools of Guy's and St Thomas's Hospitals, St Thomas' Hospital, London unpublished paper.

R.G. Bevan (1986), Problems of Financing English Acute Hospitals By Capitation, Department of Community Medicine, United Medical and Dental Schools of Guy's and St Thomas's Hospitals, St Thomas' Hospital, London, unpublished paper.

G. Bevan, R. Beech and M. Craig (1985), 'Resource allocation: alternatives to RAWP', Health and Social Service Journal, 95, 5 September, 1098-9.

R.G. Bevan and J. Brazier (1985a), 'Subregional RAWP - Hobson's choice?' Health and Social Service Journal, 95, 29 August, 1064-5.

R.G. Bevan and J. Brazier (1985b), 'Equity and efficiency: clarifying confusion for English acute hospitals', Financial Accountability and Management, 1, 173-89.

G. Bevan and J. Brazier (1986), 'Clinical incentives of sub-Regional RAWP', British Medical Journal, forthcoming.

G. Bevan and J. Charlton (1986), Reviewing RAWP: Relationships Between Resources Used by Health Authorities And General Medical Services, Department of Community Medicine, United Medical and Dental Schools of Guy's and St Thomas's Hospitals, London, unpublished paper.

G. Bevan, H. Copeman, J. Perrin and R. Rosser (1980), Health Care Priorities and Management, Croom Helm, London.

G. Bevan and R. Ingram (1986), 'Possible implications for resource allocation of inequity and its impact on clinical decisions on hospital admissions', British Medical Journal, forthcoming.

R.G. Bevan and A.H. Spencer (1984), 'Models of resource policy of Regional Health Authorities', in M. Clarke (ed) Planning and Analysis in Health Care Systems, (London Papers in Regional Science, 13) Pion, London, pp. 90-118.

S. Birch and A. Maynard (1986), The RAWP Review: RAWPing Primary Care: RAWPing the United Kingdom, Discussion Paper 19, Centre for Health Economics, University of York, York.

D.A.K. Black and J.D. Pole (1975), 'Priorities in biomedical research: Indices of burden', British Journal of Preventive and Social Medicine, 29, 222-7.

N. Bosanquet (1980), 'Health', in N. Bosanquet and P. Townsend (eds) Labour and Equality: A Fabian Study of Labour in Power 1974-79, Heinemann Educational Books, London, pp. 205-225.

A.R. Bradwell, M.H.B. Carnalt and T.P. Whitehead (1974), 'Explaining the unexpected abnormal results of biochemical profile investigations', Lancet, ii, 1071-4.

J. Brazier (1986), 'Is cross-charging a solution to the problem of cross-boundary flows?', in N. Mays, J. Brazier and R.G. Bevan Reviewing RAWP, Occasional Paper No. 1, Social Medicine and Health Services Research Unit, United Medical and Dental Schools of Guy's and St Thomas's Hospital, London.

M.E. Brennan and P.H. Clare (1980), 'The relationship between mortality and two indicators of morbidity', Journal of Epidemiology and Community Health, 34, 134-8.

M.E. Brennan and R. Lancashire (1978), 'Association of childhood mortality with housing status and unemployment', Journal of Epidemiology and Community Health, 32, 28-33.

J.R. Butler, J.M. Bevan and R.C. Taylor (1973), Family Doctors and Public Policy, Routledge and Kegan Paul, London.

M. Butts (1986), 'RAWP Review: questioning basic assumptions', The Health Service Journal, 96: 5004, 826-7.

M.S. Butts and J.R. Ashford (1977), 'A framework for planning hospital services', in G. McLachlan (ed) Framework and Design for Planning: Uses of Information in the NHS, (Problems and Progress in Medical Care: Essays on Current Research, Tenth Series), Oxford University Press for Nuffield Provincial Hospitals Trust, Oxford.

M. Butts, D. Irving and C. Whitt (1981), From Principles to Practice: A Commentary on Health Service Planning and Resource Allocation in England From 1970 to 1980, Nuffield Provincial Hospitals Trust, London.

M.J. Buxton and R.E. Klein (1975), 'Distribution of hospital provision: policy themes and resource variations', British Medical Journal, i, 345-9.

M.J. Buxton and R.E. Klein (1979), 'Population characteristics and the distribution of general medical practitioners', British Medical Journal, i, 463-66.

M. Carley (1981), Social Measurement and Social Indicators: Issues of Policy and Theory, George Allen and Unwin, London.

J.M. Carlos, G.J. Martini, B. Allen, I. Davidson and E.M. Backet (1977), 'Health indices sensitive to medical care variation', International Journal of Health Services, 7, 293-309.

J. Carrier (1978), 'Positive discrimination in the allocation of NHS resources', in M. Brown and S. Baldwin (eds) The Yearbook of Social Policy in Britain, 1977, Routledge and Kegan Paul, London, pp. 119-44.

V. Carstairs (1981), 'Multiple deprivation and health state', Community Medicine, 3, 4-13.

V. Carstairs (1982), 'Health and social deprivation', in A. Smith (ed) Recent Advances in Community Medicine 2, Churchill Livingstone, Edinburgh, pp. 51-62.

J.R.H. Charlton (1984), Medical Intervention and the Avoidability of Death, Progress Report to DHSS, Department of Community Medicine, United Medical and Dental Schools of Guy's and St Thomas's Hospitals, St Thomas' Hospital, London.

J.R.H. Charlton, R.M. Hartley, R. Silver and W.W. Holland (1983), 'Geographical variations in mortality from conditions amenable to medical intervention in England and Wales', Lancet, i, 691-6.

J.R.H. Charlton and A. Lakhani (1985), 'Is the Jarman underprivileged area score valid?', British Medical Journal, 209, 1714-6.

B.E. Coates and E.M. Rawstron (1971), Regional Variations in Britain, Batsford, London.

A.L. Cochrane (1976), 'The London hospitals' scene' [letter], British Medical Journal, ii, 1384.

College of Health (1985), Guide to Hospital Waiting Lists, The College, London, second edition.

Committee of Enquiry into the Cost of the National Health Service (1956), Report [Chairman: C.W. Guillebaud], Cmnd. 9663, HMSO, London.

M.H. Cooper (1975), Rationing Health Care, Croom Helm, London.

M.H. Cooper and A.J. Culyer (1970), 'An economic assessment of some aspects of the National Health Service', in British Medical Association Health Service Financing: A Report of the BMA Advisory Panel [Chairman: Dr I.M. Jones], Appendix A, Part IV, BMA, London.

M.H. Cooper and A.J. Culyer (1971), 'An economic survey of the nature and intent of the British National Health Service', Social Science and Medicine 5, 1-13.

M.H. Cooper and A.J. Culyer (1972), 'Equality in the National Health Service: intentions, performance and problems in evaluation', in M.M. Hauser (ed) The Economics of Medical Care, Allen and Unwin, London, pp. 47-60.

R.F. Cooper (1986), 'Are in-patient cases at a teaching hospital more difficult than District General Hospital cases?', Community Medicine, 8, 78-9.

K.M. Cottrell (1979a), 'Catchment populations: catching the drift of patient ebb and flow', Health and Social Services Journal, 12 October, 1323-4.

K.M. Cottrell (1979b), 'Out-patient survey of the North Western Region', Hospital and Health Services Review, 75, 432-4.

A.L. Creese, S.C. Darby, S.R. Palmer and D.L. Patrick (1978), 'NHS priorities and RAWP', British Medical Journal, ii, 1446-7.

R. Crossman (1977), The Diaries of A Cabinet Minister, Volume Three, Secretary of State for Social Services 1968-70, Hamish Hamilton and Jonathan Cape, London.

J.G. Cullis, D.P. Forster and C.E. Frost (1981), 'Met and unmet demand for hospital beds: some recent evidence', Revue de Epidemiologie et de Sante Publique, 29, 155-66.

A.J. Culyer and M.F. Drummond (1978), 'Financing medical education – inter-relationships between medical school and teaching hospital expenditure', in A.J. Culyer and K.G. Wright (eds) Economic Aspects of Health Services, Martin Robertson, Oxford, pp. 123-140.

A.J. Culyer, A. Maynard and A. Williams (1981), 'Alternative systems of health care provision: an essay on motes and beams', in M. Olson (ed) Health Care Regulation, American Enterprise Institute, Washington.

A.J. Culyer, J. Wiseman, M.F. Drummond and P.A. West (1978), 'What accounts for the higher costs of teaching hospitals?', Social and Economic Administration, 12, 20-30.

S. Curtis (1983), Intra-urban Variations in Health and Health Care: The Comparative Need for Health Care Survey of Tower Hamlets and Redbridge, Volume 1, Adult Morbidity and Service Use, Health Research Group, Department of Geography and Earth Sciences, Queen Mary College, London.

S. Curtis and K. Woods (1983), The Local Morbidity Survey as a Health Service Planning Instrument, paper prepared for the King Edward VII's Hospital Fund for London, Seminar, "Need for Health Services in London" held at the King's Fund Centre, London, NW1, 14 December 1983, Health Research Group, Queen Mary College, University of London, London, unpublished paper.

S.E. Curtis and K.J. Woods (1984), 'Health care in London: planning issues and the contribution of local morbidity surveys', in M. Clarke (ed) Planning and Analysis in Health Care Systems, Pion, London, pp. 57-77.

R. Dajda (1979), 'Self-reported morbidity data as an indicator of regional resource requirements', Journal of Epidemiology and Community Health, 33, 138-41.

N. Davidson (1980), 'RAWP: the honeymoon is over', Health and Social Service Journal , 90, 7 March, 320-22.

B. Davies (1968), Social Needs and Resources in Local Services, Michael Joseph, London.

R.W. Dearden (1985), Resources and Health Deprivation, HSMC Discussion Paper, 19, Health Services Management Centre, University of Birmingham, Birmingham.

W.F. Dennison (1979), 'Management developments in government resource allocation: the example of the rise and fall of P.P.B.S. (Planning-Programming-Budgeting-System)', Journal of Management Studies, October, 220-82.

Departments of the Environment and Transport (undated), The Airport Inquiries 1981-1983, Extracts from the report of the Inspector, Graham Eyre QC, Departments of the Environment and Transport, London.

DHSS (1970a), The Future of the National Health Service, HMSO, London. (2nd Green Paper).

DHSS (1970b), Hospital Revenue Allocations, Paper RHB Chairmen 3/70, DHSS, London, unpublished.

DHSS (1972a), Management Arrangements for the Reorganised National Health Service, HMSO, London.

DHSS (1972b), National Health Service Reorganisation: England, Cmnd 5055, HMSO, London.

DHSS (1973),   Health Service Reorganisation Circular, HRC(73)3, DHSS, London.

DHSS (1975),   Regional Resource Allocation Formula: First Interim Report of the RAWP, DHSS, London.

DHSS (1976a),   Priorities for Health and Personal Social Services in England: A Consultative Document, HMSO, London.

DHSS (1976b),   Regional Planning Guidelines, 1976-77, HC(76)29, DHSS, London.

DHSS (1976c),   Sharing Resources for Health in England, Report of the Resource Allocation Working Party, HMSO, London.

DHSS (1976d),   Relationship Between SMRs and Other Indicators of Deprivation, Paper prepared by DHSS (SR4A), DHSS, London, unpublished.

DHSS (1977a),   Priorities in the Health and Personal Social Services: The Way Forward, HMSO, London.

DHSS (1977b),   A Classification of the English Personal Social Services Authorities (by Valerie Imber), DHSS Statistical and Research Report Series, No. 16, HMSO, London.

DHSS (1978),   RAWP and the National Programme Budget: Report of the Procedures and Costing Sub-Group of the Standing Group on NHS Planning, SGP (78)24, DHSS, London, unpublished paper.

DHSS (1979),   Patients First:Consultative Paper on the Structure and Management of the National Health Service in England and Wales, HMSO, London.

DHSS (1980a),   Inequalities in Health: Report of a Research Working Group (Chairman: Sir Douglas Black), DHSS, London.

DHSS (1980b),   Report of the Advisory Group on Resource Allocation, DHSS, London.

DHSS (1981),   Care in Action: A Handbook of Policies and Priorities for the Health and Personal Social Services in England, HMSO, London.

DHSS (1983),   Report of the NHS Management Inquiry (Leader: Roy Griffiths), DHSS, London, mimeo.

DHSS (1984a),   Proposed Changes to RAWP Target Calculations, Paper RT/84/16, DHSS, London, unpublished.

DHSS (1984b),   Final Report of the Acute Services Working Group of the Joint Group on Performance Indicators, DHSS, London.

DHSS (1985a),   Performance Indicators for the NHS 1983/4. DHSS, London, computer discs.

DHSS (1985b),   Hospital and Community Health Services, 1985-86 Cash limits: Exposition Booklet, DHSS-FA2B, DHSS, London.

DHSS (1985c),   The Health Service in England, Annual Report 1985, HMSO, London.

DHSS (1986a),   Review of the RAWP Formula (Letter from the Chairman of the NHS Management Board, Victor Paige, to consultees), NHS Management Board, DHSS, London.

DHSS (1986b),   Performance Indicators for the NHS, 1984/5, DHSS, London, computer discs.

DHSS and Thames Regional Health Authorities (1979), Assessing Target Allocations Within the Thames Regions: Report of a Joint Working Group, DHSS, London.

R. Dowie (1978),   'Demographic and socio-economic indices and sickness absence statistics: their relevance as morbidity indicators', in J. Brotherston (ed) Morbidity and Its Relationship to Resource Allocation, Welsh Office, Cardiff, pp. 43–96.

R. Dowie (1985),   Allowances for Social Deprivation in the South West Thames Sub-Regional RAWP Formula, Unpublished report to St George's Hospital Medical School.

R. Dredge (1984),   'Diagnosis related groups: how DRGs can help with the budget', Health and Social Service Journal, 94, 2 August, 918–19.

H.A.F. Dudley (1977),   'Loosening patient immobility', Lancet, i, 1251–3.

J. Edwards (1975),   'Social indicators, urban deprivation and positive discrimination', Journal of Social Policy, 4, 275–87.

H. Elcock and S. Haywood (1980), The Buck Stops Where? Accountability and Control in the National Health Service', Institute for Health Studies, University of Hull, Hull.

A.C. Enthoven (1985a),   Reflections on the Management of the National Health Service: An American Looks at Incentives to Efficiency in Health Services Management in the UK, Nuffield Provincial Hospitals Trust, London.

A.C. Enthoven (1985b),   The US Health Care Economy: From Guild to Market in Ten Years, Graduate School of Business, Stanford University, Stanford.

J. Eyles, D.M. Smith and K.J. Woods (1982), 'Spatial resource allocation and state practice: the case of health service planning in London', Regional Studies, 16, 239–53.

J. Feinmann (1985),   'Plan to shop around for operations is torpedoed', Health and Social Service Journal, 95, 21 February, 213.

M.S. Feldstein (1965),   'Hospital bed scarcity: an analysis of the effects of inter-regional differences', Economica, 32, 393–409.

M.S. Feldstein (1967),   Economic Analysis of Health Service Efficiency, North Holland Publishing Company, Amsterdam.

H.P. Ferrer, A. Moore and G.C. Stevens (1977), 'The use of mortality data in the report of the Resource Allocation Working Party (HMSO, 1976)', Public Health, Lon., 91, 289-95.

R.B. Fetter, Y. Shin, J.L. Freeman, R.F. Averill and J.D. Thompson (1980), 'Case mix definition by diagnosis-related groups', Medical Care (suppl.), 18, 1-53.

R.B. Fetter, R.F. Averill, J.F. Lichtenstein and J.L. Freeman (undated), Ambulatory Visit Groups: A Framework for Measuring Productivity in Ambulatory Care, Health Systems Management Group, School of Organisation and Management, Yale University, New Haven, Conneticett.

G.R. Ford (1972), 'Comment on "Equality in the National Health Service: intentions, performance and problems in evaluation"', in M.M. Hauser (ed) The Economics of Medical Care, Allen and Unwin, London, pp. 58-60.

D.P. Forster (1977), 'Mortality, morbidity and resource allocation', Lancet, i, 997-8.

D.P. Forster (1978), 'Mortality as an indicator of morbidity in resource allocation', in J. Brotherston (ed) Morbidity and its Relationship to Resource Allocation, Welsh Office, Cardiff, pp. 13-24.

D.P. Forster (1979), 'The relationships between health needs, socio-environmental indices, general practitioner resources and utilisation', Journal of Chronic Disease, 32, 333-7.

G. Forsyth and R.M. Varley (1981), 'Health and the Inner City Partnerships: an experiment in collaboration', in G. McLachlan (ed) Matters of Moment (Problems and Progress in Medical Care, Essays on Current Research, 13th series), Nuffield Provincial Hospitals Trust, London, pp. 41-69.

J.M. Forsythe, W.W. Holland, A.J. Lane, A.E. Bennett and A.H. Snaith (1976), 'The London hospitals' scene' [Letter], British Medical Journal, ii, 1320.

A.J. Fox and P.O. Goldblatt (1982), Longitudinal Study: Socio-demographic Mortality Differentials 1971-75, Series L5, No.1, OPCS, London.

A.J. Fox, D.R. Jones and P.O. Goldblatt (1984), 'Approaches to studying the effect of socio-economic circumstances on geographic differences in mortality in England and Wales', British Medical Bulletin, 40: 4, 309-14.

P.D. Fox (1978), 'Managing health resources: English style', in G. McLachlan (ed) By Guess or by What? Information Without Design in the NHS, Nuffield Provincial Hospitals Trust, London, pp. 3-64.

R.J. Gandy (1979a), 'A comparison of two proxy measures for morbidity', Journal of Epidemiology and Community Health, 33, 100-3.

R.J. Gandy (1979b),   'The calculation of catchment populations within the National Health Service', Statistician, 28: 1, 29-37.

M.J. Gardner, P.D. Winter and D.J.P. Barker (1984), Atlas of Mortality from Selected Diseases, John Wiley, Chichester.

K. Geary (1977),   'Technical deficiencies in RAWP', British Medical Journal, i, 1367.

P.H. Gentle and J.M. Forsythe (1975), 'Revenue allocation in the reorganized health service', British Medical Journal, iii, 382-4.

J. Gibson and T. Travers (1985), 'Block grant: the story of a failure', Public Money, 5:2, 17-22.

H. Glennerster (1981), 'From containment to conflict? Social planning in the seventies', Journal of Social Policy, 10, 31-51.

Sir G. Godber (1975),   'Regional devolution and the National Health Service', in E. Craven (ed) Regional Devolution and Social Policy, Macmillan/Centre for Studies in Social Policy, London, pp. 59-85.

M.J. Goldacre (1981),   'Mortality statistics as measures of need for outpatient services', British Medical Journal, 283, 870-1.

M.J. Goldacre and R.I. Harris (1980), 'Mortality, morbidity, resource allocation and planning: a consideration of disease classification', British Medical Journal, 281, 1515-9.

A.M. Gray and D.J. Hunter (1983), 'Priorities and resource allocation in the Scottish health service: some problems in 'planning and implementation'', Policy and Politics, 11, 417-37.

A. Gray and G. Mooney (1981), Scotland's Health and Health Care, Health Economics Research Unit Discussion Paper No. 11/81, Health Economics Research Unit, Departments of Community Medicine and Political Economy, University of Aberdeen, Aberdeen.

Greater London Council Health Panel (1984), A Critical Guide to Health Service Resource Allocation in London, Greater London Council, London.

G. Greenshields (1984), 'Learning to live with cash limits - and other financial matters', British Medical Journal, 288, 1393-95.

D.A.T. Griffiths (1971), 'Inequalities and management in the NHS', The Hospital, July, 229-233.

S. Halpern (1985),   'Management: how should the centre be spread?', Health and Social Service Journal, 95, 28 February, 248-50.

C. Ham (1981),   Policy-making in the National Health Service: A Case Study of the Leeds Regional Hospital Board, Macmillan, London.

C. Ham (1985),   Health Policy in Britain, Macmillan, London, second edition.

J.T. Hart (1971),   'The inverse care law', Lancet, i, 405-412.

S. Haywood (1983),   'The politics of management in health care: a British perspective,' Journal of Health Politics, Policy and Law, 8, 424-43.

S. Haywood and A. Alaszewski (1980), Crisis in the Health Service, Croom Helm, London.

S. Haywood and J. Yates (1986), 'London's unhealthy appetite', The Times, Friday 5 September.

M.A. Heasman (1979),   'Measurement of morbidity for resource allocation - a discussion paper', Health Bulletin, 37: 4, 103-7.

T. Heller (1979),   'Rural health and health services', in J.M. Shaw (ed) Rural Deprivation and Planning, Geo Abstracts/University of East Anglia, Norwich, pp. 81-92.

C. Hodges (1986),   'North Western - a region that has lost its way', The Health Service Journal, 96: 5023, 1414-5.

W.W. Holland (1984),   'Teaching hospitals in crisis: expensive luxury or vital asset?', Lancet, ii, 742-43.

W.W. Holland (1986),   'The RAWP review: pious hopes', Lancet, ii, 1087-90.

W.W. Holland, J. Charlton, D.L. Patrick and P.A. West (1980), The RAWP Project, Department of Community Medicine, St Thomas's Hospital Medical School, London.

J.R. Hollingsworth (1981), 'Inequalities in levels of health in England and Wales, 1891-1971', Journal of Health and Social Behavior, 22, 268-83.

D. Holmes (1984),   'Out patient referrals', Health and Social Service Journal, 94: 4923, 4-6.

S. Horn, P.D. Starkey and D.A. Bertram (1983), 'Measuring severity of illness: homogeneous case mix groups', Medical Care, 21:1, 14-30.

House of Commons Expenditure Committee (1971), Memorandum Submitted by DHSS to the House of Commons Expenditure Committee (Employment and Social Services Sub-Committee), Session 1970/71, Minutes of Evidence, Wednesday, 31 March 1971, HMSO, London.

House of Commons Public Accounts Committee (1981), Financial Control and Accountability in the NHS, Seventeenth Report from the Public Accounts Committee, Session 1980-81, (HC 255) HMSO, London.

House of Commons Public Accounts Committee (1982), Financial Control and Accountability in the NHS, Seventeenth Report from the Public Accounts Committee, Session 1981-82, (HC 375) HMSO, London.

G.M. Howe (1963),   National Atlas of Mortality in the United Kingdom, Nelson, London.

S. Hunt and J. McEwen   (1980), 'The development of a subjective health indicator', <u>Sociology of Health and Illness</u>, 2, 231-46.

D.J. Hunter (1980),   <u>Coping with Uncertainty: Policy and Politics in the National Health Service</u>, Research Studies Press/Wiley and Sons, Chichester.

D. Hunter (1983),   'Patterns of organisation for health: a systems overview of the National Health Service in the United Kingdom', in A. Williamson and G. Room (eds) <u>Health and Welfare States of Britain: an Inter-country Comparison</u>, Heinemann Education Books, London, pp. 56-88.

J.K. Iglehart (1982),   'The new era of prospective payment for hospitals', <u>New England Journal of Medicine</u>, 307: 20, 1288-92.

D. Irving (1983a),   <u>Identification of Underprivileged Areas: Measuring the Need for NHS Services in the Community</u>, Technical Paper, London School of Economics and Political Science, London.

D. Irving (1983b),   'Areas of deprivation: how statistics can plot areas of need', <u>Health and Social Service Journal</u>, 93, 1262-3.

D. Irving (1985),   'How to identify the needy', <u>Health and Social Service Journal</u>, 95, 18-19.

B. Jarman (1983),   'Identification of underprivileged areas', <u>British Medical Journal</u>, 286, 705-9.

B. Jarman (1984),   'Underprivileged areas: validation and distribution of scores', <u>British Medical Journal</u>, 289, 1587-92.

B. Jarman (1985),   'Underprivileged areas', in D.J. Pereira Gray (ed) <u>The Medical Annual 1985</u>, Wright, Bristol, pp. 224-43.

M. Jeffries (1978),   'RAWP and the Oxford Region', <u>British Medical Journal</u>, i, 426-7, 495-6 and 638-9.

L. Jenkins and J. Coles (1984), 'Diagnosis related groups: information tools for the future', <u>Health and Social Service Journal</u>, 94, 9 August, 948-9.

D.R. Jones and A. Bourne (1975), 'The distribution of resources in the National Health Service', <u>Hospital and Health Services Review</u>, 71, 382-4.

D.R. Jones and A. Bourne (1976), 'Monitoring the distribution of resources in the National Health Service', <u>Social and Economic Administration</u>, 10, 92-105.

D.R. Jones and S. Masterman (1976), 'NHS resources: scales of variation', <u>British Journal of Preventive and Social Medicine</u>, 30, 244-50.

T. Jones and M. Prowle (1984), <u>Health Service Finance: An Introduction</u>, Certified Accountants' Educational Trust, London, second edition.

S.J. Kilpatrick (1963) 'Mortality comparisons in socio-economic groups', <u>Applied Statistics</u>, 12, 65-86.

R. Klein (1974),   'Policy making in the National Health Service', Political Studies, 22:1, 1-14.

R. Klein (1975),   'The National Health Service', in R. Klein (ed) Inflation and Priorities: Social Policy and Public Expenditure, 1975, Centre for Studies in Social Policy, London, pp. 83-104.

R. Klein (1976),   'The politics of redistribution', British Medical Journal, ii, 893-5.

R.E.Klein (1977),   'Resource allocation', Hospital and Health Services Review, 73: 8, 280-4.

R. Klein (1979),   'Ideology, class and The National Health Service', Journal of Health Politics, Policy and Law, 4:3, 464-90.

R. Klein (1981),   'The strategy behind the Jenkin non-strategy', British Medical Journal, 282, 1089-91.

R. Klein (1983),   The Politics of the National Health Service, Longman, London.

R. Klein and M. Buxton (1974), 'Health inequities', New Society, 7 November, 357-8.

E.G. Knox, T. Marshall, S. Kane, A. Green and R. Mallett (1980), 'Social and health care determinants of area variations in perinatal mortality', Community Medicine, 2, 282-90.

P.L. Knox (1978),   'The intraurban ecology of primary medical care: patterns of accessibility and their policy implications', Environment and Planning A, 10, 415-35.

P.L. Knox (1979),   'Medical deprivation, area deprivation and public policy', Social Science and Medicine, 13D, 111-21.

P.L. Knox (1981),   'Convergence and divergence in Regional patterns of infant mortality in the United Kingdom from 1949-51 to 1970-72', Social Science and Medicine, 15D, 323-8.

M. Lally (1980),   'Resource allocation in London's health service: a note', Greater London Intelligence Journal, no. 44,33-4.

R.J. Lavers and M. Rees (1972), 'The Distinction Award system in England and Wales', in G. McLachlan (ed) Problems and Progress in Medical Care, 7th series, NPHT, London.

R. Leavey and J. Wood (1985), 'Does the underprivileged area index work?', British Medical Journal, 291, 709-11.

K. Lee (1977),   'Public expenditure, planning and local democracy', in K. Barnard and K. Lee (eds) Conflicts in the National Health Service, Croom Helm, London, pp. 210-31.

K. Lee (1982),   'Public expenditure, health services and health', in A. Walker (ed) Public Expenditure and Social Policy: An Examination of Social Spending and Social Priorities, Heinemann Education Books, London, pp. 73-90.

R.F.L. Logan, J.S.A. Ashley, R.E. Klein and D.M. Robson (1972), Dynamics of Medical Care: The Liverpool Study Into Use of Hospital Resources, Department of Community Health, London School of Hygiene and Tropical Medicine, Memoir No. 14, London School of Hygiene and Tropical Medicine, London.

London Health Planning Consortium (1979), Acute Hospital Services in London: A Profile by the London Health Planning Consortium, HMSO, London.

London Health Planning Consortium (1980), Towards A Balance: A Framework for Acute Hospital Services in London Reconciling Service with Teaching Needs, HMSO, London.

London Health Planning Consortium (1981), Primary Health Care in Inner London: Report of a Study Commissioned by the LHPC, (The Acheson Report) LHPC, London.

A. Ludbrook and A. Maynard (1983), 'The Regional allocation of health care resources in the UK and France', Social Policy And Administration, 17, 232-248.

M. McCarthy (1986), 'A fairer deal from RAWP', British Medical Journal, 292, 289-290.

S. McIntyre (1986), 'The patterning of health by social position in contemporary Britain: directions for sociological research', Social Science and Medicine, 23: 4, 393-415.

K. McPherson, P. Strong, A. Epstein and L. Jones (1981), 'Regional variations in the use of common surgical procedures: within and between, England and Wales, Canada and the United States of America', Social Science and Medicine, 15A, 273-88.

W.G. Manning, A. Liebowitz, G.A. Goldberg, W.H. Rogers and J.P. Newhouse (1984), 'A controlled trial of the effect of a pre-paid group practice on use of services', New England Journal of Medicine, 310, 1505-10.

M.G. Marmot, A.M. Adelstein and L. Bulusu (1984), Immigrant Mortality in England and Wales 1970-78: Causes of Death by Country of Birth, OPCS Studies on Medical and Population Subjects, no. 47, HMSO, London.

R. Maxwell (1984), 'Costs of teaching hospitals', British Medical Journal, 289, 714-5.

J.J. May (ed) (1982), 'Diagnosis related groups', Topics in Health Care Financing, 8, 1-81.

A. Maynard (1972), 'Inequalities in psychiatric care in England and Wales', Social Science and Medicine, 6, 221-7.

A. Maynard and A. Ludbrook (1980a), 'Budget allocation in the National Health Service', Journal of Social Policy, 9, 289-312.

A. Maynard and A. Ludbrook (1980b), 'What's wrong with The National Health Service?', Lloyd's Bank Review, no. 138, October, 27-41.

A. Maynard and A. Ludbrook (1980c), 'Applying resource allocation formulae to constituent parts of the UK', Lancet , i, 85-7.

A. Maynard and A. Ludbrook (1982), 'Inequality, the National Health Service and health policy', Journal of Public Policy , 2, 97-116.

A. Maynard and A. Ludbrook (1983), 'The allocation of health care resources in the United Kingdom', in A. Williamson and G. Room (eds) Health and Welfare States of Britain: An Inter-Country Comparison , Heinemann Education Books, London, pp. 89-106.

A. Maynard and R. Tingle (1976), 'The objectives and performance of the mental health services in England and Wales in the 1960s', Journal of Social Policy , 4, 151-168.

N. Mays (1986), 'SMRs, social deprivation or what?', in N. Mays, J. Brazier and R.G. Bevan Reviewing RAWP, Occasional Paper No. 1, Social Medicine and Health Services Research Unit, United Medical and Dental Schools of Guy's and St Thomas's Hospitals, St Thomas' Hospital, London.

Mersey Regional Health Authority (1983), SMRs, Morbidity and Deprivation, Document ORS 83/2, Mersey RHA Operational Research and Statistics Section, Mersey RHA, Liverpool.

R. Milner, I.S. Johnson, M. Watts, A.I. Coupland, A.M. Coyne and J.N. Todd (1986), 'On the state of health in inner cities' [letter], British Medical Journal, 292, 1276.

Ministry of Health (1944), A National Health Service , Cmnd. 6502, HMSO, London.

Ministry of Health (1946), The National Health Service Bill: A Summary of the Proposed Service , Cmnd. 6761, HMSO, London.

Ministry of Health (1962), A Hospital Plan for England and Wales, Cmnd 1604, HMSO, London.

Ministry of Health (1966), The Hospital Building Programme: A Revision of the Hospital Plan for England and Wales, Cmnd. 3000, HMSO, London.

G. Mooney (1984), 'Programme budgeting: an aid to planning and priority setting in health care', Effective Health Care , 2, 65-8.

G.H. Mooney, E.M. Russell and R.D. Weir (1980), Choices for Health Care, Macmillan, London.

M. Morgan (1983), 'Measuring social inequality: occupational classifications and their alternatives', Community Medicine , 5, 116-24.

M. Morgan and S. Chinn (1983), 'ACORN group, social class and child health', Journal of Epidemiology and Community Health , 37, 196-203.

J.N Morris (1976), Uses of Epidemiology, Churchill Livingstone, Edinburgh.

K. Morris (1979),   'Resource allocation: blueprint for the brave new world', Health and Social Service Journal, 89, 24 August, 1079-80.

P. Mullen (1978),   RAWP and Resource Allocation in the NHS, Health Services Management Centre Occasional Paper 23, University of Birmingham, Health Services Management Centre, Birmingham.

National Association of Health Authorities (1983), The Sub-Regional Application of RAWP by Regional Health Authorities, NAHA, Birmingham.

National Association of Health Authorities (1986), Fair Shares In The NHS: NAHA's Evidence to the NHS Management Board's Review of RAWP, NAHA, Birmingham.

NHS/DHSS Steering Group on Health Services Information (1984a), The Collection and Use of Information About Activity in Hospitals and the Community, Fourth Report to the Secretary of State, (Chairman: Mrs E Korner), HMSO, London.

NHS/DHSS Steering Group on Health Services Information (1984b), A Report on the Collection and Use of Financial Information in the National Health Service, Sixth Report to the secretary of State, (Chairman: Mrs E Korner), HMSO, London.

North East Thames Regional Health Authority (1983a), Patient Census Study: Social Factor Analysis , NETRHA Management Services Report No. 1249, NETRHA, London.

North East Thames Regional Health Authority (1983b), Further Analysis of Patient Census Data with Respect to Social Deprivation , NETRHA Management Services Report No. 1259, NETRHA, London.

North West Thames Regional Health Authority (undated), Hospital Inpatient Census 1981: Analysis of the Data, NWTRHA, London.

North West Thames Regional Health Authority (1984a), Towards A Strategy for Acute Services, NWTRHA, London.

North West Thames Regional Health Authority (1984b), 1984/85 Sub-Regional RAWP Targets , Regional Treasurer's Department, NWTRHA, London.

J. Noyce, A.H. Snaith and A.J. Trickey (1974), 'Regional variations in the allocation of financial resources to the community health services', Lancet, i, 554-7.

Nuffield Provincial Hospitals Trust (1946), The Hospital Surveys: The Domesday Book of the Hospital Service, Oxford University Press, London.

Office of Population Censuses and Surveys (1978), Occupational Mortality Decennial Supplement, 1970-72 , Series DS No. 1, HMSO, London.

Office of Population Censuses and Surveys (1983), Mid-1981 Based Sub-National Population Projections for England, OPCS Monitor, PP 3 83/1, OPCS, London.

D. Owen (1976),   In Sickness and in Health: The Politics of Medicine, Quartet Books, London.

S.R. Palmer (1978),   'The use of mortality data in resource allocation', in J. Brotherston (ed) Morbidity and Its Relationship to Resource Allocation, Welsh Office, Cardiff, pp. 25-39.

S. Palmer, P. West and P.   Dodd (1980), 'Randomness in the RAWP formula: the reliability of mortality data in the allocation of National Health Service revenue', Journal of Epidemiology and Community Health, 34, 212-6.

S. Palmer, P. West, D. Patrick and M.   Glynn (1979), 'Mortality indices in resource allocation', Community Medicine, 1, 275-81.

C. Paton (1985),   The Policy of Resource Allocation and Its Ramifications: A Review, Nuffield Provincial Hospitals Trust, London.

D. Patrick, W. Holland, S. Palmer and P.   West (1980), 'On measuring need for health service resources', in W.W.   Holland, J. Charlton, D.L.   Patrick and P.A.   West The RAWP Project , Social Medicine and Health Services Research Unit, St Thomas's Hospital Medical School, London, mimeo, Appendix D.

J.R. Perrin and M. Magee (1982), The Costs, Joint Products and Funding of English Teaching Hospitals , Warwick Papers in Industry, Business and Administration, no.   8, University of Warwick, Centre for Research in Industry, Business and Administration, School of Industrial and Business Studies, Coventry.

D.C. Pinder (1982),   'Catchment populations: the properties and accuracy of various methods for their estimation', Community Medicine, 4, 188-195.

D.C. Pinder (1985),   'Weighting populations for their mortality experience', Community Medicine, 7, 107-115.

C. Pollitt (1984),   'Case study: inequalities in health care', in Open University Social Sciences, a Third Level Course: Social Policy and Social Welfare - Block 4, Case Studies in British Social Policy, Units 11, 12 and 13, (D355/4 (11,12 & 13)) Open University Press, Milton Keynes, pp. 37-84.

Radical Statistics Health Group (1977), RAW(P) Deals: A Critique of "Sharing Resources for Health in England" (the RAWP Report), Radical Statistics Health Group, London, mimeo.

T. Richardson (1984), 'Under the banyan tree', Lancet, i, 727-8.

J.H. Rickard (1974),   The Allocation of Revenue Expenditure Between Areas in the Reorganised Health Service , University of Oxford, Department of the Regius Professor of Medicine, Oxford.

J.H. Rickard (1976),   'Per capita expenditure of the English Area Health Authorities', British Medical Journal , i, 299-300.

V.G. Rodwin (1984),   The Health Planning Predicament: France, Quebec, England and the United States, University of California Press, Berkeley.

Royal Commission on the National Health Service (1978a), Management of Financial Resources in the National Health Service, Research Paper No. 2, (By J. Perrin et al) HMSO, London.

Royal Commission on the National Health Service (1978b), Allocating Health Resources: A Commentary on the Report of the Resource Allocation Working Party, Research Paper No. 3, (By M.J. Buxton and R.E. Klein) HMSO, London.

Royal Commission on the National Health Service (1979), Report, (Chairman: Sir A. Merrison) Cmnd. 7615, HMSO, London.

C. Sanderson (1979),   Sharing Revenue Funds Within and Between Health Authorities: Services for Non-Psychiatric Inpatients, (A paper for the Committee of Area Specialists in Community Medicine (Information), East Anglian RHA) University of Cambridge, Department of Community Medicine, Cambridge, unpublished paper.

H.F. Sanderson, M. Craig, G.P.A. Winyard and R.G. Bevan (1986), 'Using Diagnosis-Related Groups in the NHS', Community Medicine, 8:1, 37-46.

Scottish Home and Health Department (1977), Scottish Health Authorities Revenue Equalisation (SHARE): Report of the Working Party on Revenue Resource Allocation, HMSO, Edinburgh.

A. Scott-Samuel (1977), 'Social area analysis in community medicine', British Journal of Preventive and Social Medicine, 31, 199-204.

A. Scott-Samuel (1984), 'Need for primary health care: an objective indicator', British Medical Journal, 288, 457-8.

S.J. Senn and H. Shaw (1978), 'Resource allocation: some problems in applying the national formula to area and district revenue allocations', Journal of Epidemiology and Community Health, 22, 32-37.

A. Shonfield and S. Shaw (eds) (1972), Social Indicators and Social Policy, Heinemann for SSRC, London.

A. Skrimshire (1978),   Area Disadvantage, Social Class and the Health Service, (A Pilot Study of Variation Between Areas in Reported Sickness and in the Experience of Receiving General Practice Care), University of Oxford, Social Evaluation Unit, Department of Social and Administrative Studies, Oxford, in association with Canning Town Community Development Project.

J. Smith (1984),   'Hospital building in the NHS: Policy I', British Medical Journal, 289, 1298-1300.

J.C.C. Smith (1986),   'RAWP revisited', THS Health Summary, in press.

A.H. Snaith (1978), 'Subregional resource allocations in the National Health Service', Journal of Epidemiology and Community Health, 32, 16-21.

Social Medicine and Health Services Research Unit and Division of Community Health (1985), Progress Report 1980-1985, United Medical and Dental Schools of Guy's and St Thomas's Hospitals, St Thomas' Campus, London.

South East Thames Regional Health Authority (1985), ACORN and RAWP: An Allowance for Social Deprivation, Statistics and Operational Research Department, South East Thames RHA, Bexhill-on-Sea.

South East Thames Regional Health Authority (1986a), ACORN: An Allowance for Social Factors in RAWP, Consultative Paper, Statistics and Operational Research Division, South East Thames RHA, Bexhill-on-Sea.

South East Thames Regional Health Authority (1986b), Regional Review: Contracting Out Between Health Authorities, Report prepared for the Regional Chairmen's Group, South East Thames RHA, Bexhill-on-Sea.

V. Speller and D. Hale (1985), 'Making the most of your postcode', Health and Social Service Journal, 95: 4937, 252-3.

Q. Thompson and M. Lally (1980), 'London's health services: an overview', in M. McCarthy (ed) London's Health Services in the 80s, King's Fund Project Paper 25/1, King's Fund Centre, London, pp. 38-59.

C. Thunhurst (1985), 'The analysis of small area statistics and planning for health', The Statistician, 34, 93-106.

P. Townsend, P. Phillimore and A. Beattie (1986), Inequalities In Health In The Northern Region: An Interim Report, Northern Regional Health Authority and University of Bristol, Newcastle-upon-Tyne and Bristol.

P. Townsend, D. Simpson and N. Tibbs (1984), Inequalities in Health in the City of Bristol: A Preliminary Review of Statistical Evidence, University of Bristol, Department of Social Administration, Bristol.

R. Varley (1982), Understanding Resource Allocation in the NHS – the Development of RAWP, University of Manchester, Health Services Management Unit, Manchester.

G.J.A. Walker (1978), Re-allocation of Resources: The Need for More Appropriate Information on Relative Need, Paper for the North East Thames Health Information Group, London School of Hygiene and Tropical Medicine, London, unpublished.

R. Weeden (1980), Geographic Variations in the Cost of Health Service Inputs, Economic Advisers' Office, DHSS, London.

Wessex Regional Health Authority (1984), <u>Wessex Regional Plan, 1984</u>, Wessex RHA, Winchester.

P.A. West (1973),   'Allocation and equity in the public sector: the Hospital Revenue Allocation Formula', <u>Applied Economics</u>, 5, 153-66.

P. West (1976),   'Equity in health service provision: the formula approach', <u>Social and Economic Administration</u>, 10, 83-91.

P.A. West, S.R. Palmer, D. Patrick and P. Dodd (1980), 'Sharing fairly in the NHS: the effect of imperfect cost data in RAWP', <u>Hospital and Health Services Review</u>, 76:10, 330-4.

R. West (1978),   'Bed usage and disease specific mortality within ICD chapters', <u>Journal of Epidemiology and Community Health</u>, 32, 38-40.

R.R. West and C.R. Lowe (1976), 'Regional variations in need for and provision of and use of child health services in England and Wales', <u>British Medical Journal</u>, ii, 843-6.

W.F. Whimster (1976), 'Personal view', <u>British Medical Journal</u>, ii, 1318.
A. Wildavsky (1974), <u>The Politics of the Budgetary Process</u>, Little Brown, Boston.

D. Wilkin, D.H.M. Metcalfe, L. Hallam, M. Cooke and P.K. Hodgkin (1984), 'Area variations in the process of care in urban general practice', <u>British Medical Journal</u>, 289: 6439, 229-32.

G.P.A. Winyard (1981), 'RAWP - new injustice for old?' <u>British Medical Journal</u>, 283, 930-2.

J. Wood (1983),   'Are the problems of primary care in inner cities fact or fiction?', <u>British Medical Journal</u>, 286, 1109-12.

P.W. Wood (1984),   <u>Geographical Equity and Inpatient Hospital Care: An Empirical Analysis</u>, HERU Discussion Paper No. 05/84, University of Aberdeen, Departments of Community Medicine and Political Economy, Health Economics Research Unit, Aberdeen.

K.J. Woods (1982),   'Social deprivation and resource allocation in the Thames Regional Health Authorities', In Health Research Group <u>Contemporary Perspectives on Health and Health Care</u>, Occasional Paper No. 20, University of London, Queen Mary College, Department of Geography and Earth Science, London.